obesity

and weight management in primary care

"From Samoa to the Steppes, from Sao Paolo to Sydney – every country faces a potential public health disaster if it fails to take decisive measures not only to introduce better management but far more effective preventive measures to halt the slide we have seen accelerating over the past 25 years".

Professor W.P.T. James
Chairman, International Obesity Task Force, 1999

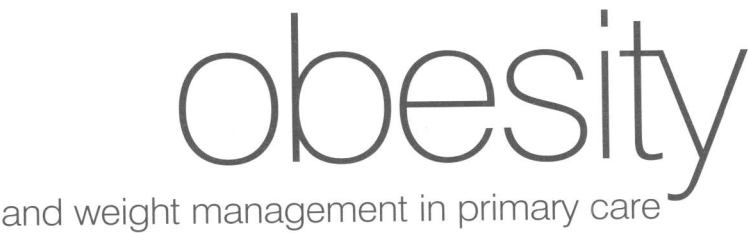

obesity
and weight management in primary care

Colin Waine OBE, FRCGP, FRCPath
Director of Health Programmes and
Primary Care Development
Sunderland Health Authority
Sunderland, UK

Foreword by
Nick Bosanquet
Professor of Health Policy
Imperial College
London, UK

Blackwell
Science

© 2002 by Blackwell Science Ltd
a Blackwell Publishing Company
EDITORIAL OFFICES:
Osney Mead, Oxford OX2 0EL, UK
  Tel: +44 (0)1865 206206
Blackwell Science, Inc., 350 Main Street, Malden, MA 02148-5018, USA
  Tel: +1 781 388 8250
Blackwell Science Asia Pty, 54 University Street, Carlton, Victoria 3053, Australia
  Tel: +61 (0)3 9347 0300
Blackwell Wissenschafts Verlag, Kurfürstendamm 57, 10707 Berlin, Germany
  Tel: +49 (0)30 32 79 060

First published 2002

Catalogue records for this title are available from the British Library and Library of Congress

ISBN 0-632-06514-1

Set in 9/11.5pt Sabon
Text layout and design by Designers Collective Limited
Printed and bound in Great Britain by Ashford Colour Press Ltd, Gosport, Hants.

For further information on Blackwell Science, visit our website:
www.blackwell-science.co.uk

Contents

Foreword

Risk factor is a term which strikes uneasily at the conscience of health professionals. In socially deprived areas almost every second patient bears witness to the possible impact of risk factors such as obesity and smoking on their health and even survival: but in the pressure of day-to-day consultations there is rarely time to do more than treat symptoms rather than deal with causes. Dr Colin Waine writes from experience as a GP and as a leader in primary care programmes. He is one of a small group of innovators from the North East who have influenced primary care in the region and well beyond it.

Obesity and Weight Management in Primary Care is a useful summary of the evidence on the disease of obesity which impacts both on quality of life and on ill health. The text gives a careful review of the links to long-term illness, especially diabetes and cardiovascular disease. It also sets realistic targets for making a difference. There is no need to aim for ideal weight – even a reduction of 5–10 kilos could make a real difference in reducing later ill health.

The problem remains how this is to be a priority in a world where the short-term and the urgent press in. There has to be realistic recognition of the time and effort required to get results in this field and this is where Dr Waine's book goes beyond a review of the evidence. He sets out a practical programme for a PCO based on a specialist centre for weight management which stresses communication and the shared setting of goals as well as a detailed programme for diet and exercise. He also sets out the potentially valuable role of new drug therapies in adding to the range of options for effective programmes.

In 1996 16 per cent of men and 18 per cent of women were obese – and with change in diet and more sedentary lifestyle the problem is set to get worse. Dr Waine also provides evidence on childhood obesity and on economic costs of obesity. He has set the item firmly on the agenda for PCOs and PCTs.

Nick Bosanquet
Professor of Health Policy,
Imperial College, London

Preface

Obesity is undoubtedly the major nutritional disorder of the western world. In fact, it has such a major impact on mortality, morbidity and quality of life that it most certainly merits consideration as a disease in its own right.

All western nations are facing a burgeoning of the problems associated with obesity. The UK, for example, is facing a veritable epidemic as the prevalence doubled between 1980 and 1991. While the bad news is that the prevalence of obesity is rising, the good news is that achieving and maintaining relatively modest weight loss can have a major beneficial impact of the risk of developing those common and life-threatening conditions such as type 2 diabetes, ischaemic heart disease and certain cancers of which it is so often the precursor.

Obesity is not just a matter of gluttony or sloth; it results from complex interactions between genetic and environmental factors, some of which are beyond conscious individual human control.

If we are really intent on improving the health of the nation, then halting the current epidemic of obesity must be high on our agenda. To do so will require a combination of public health and individual approaches and the obvious place for the latter is primary care.

In this book I have tried to emphasize the importance of taking obesity seriously – as a disease in its own right and of managing it as such.

The fact that we no longer need to strive for the well nigh unachievable goal of ideal body weight should make the task of tackling obesity less daunting for both patients and professionals. Hopefully, what follows will help them to success.

Acknowledgements

My grateful thanks to Professor W.P.T. James for permission to include material from his article 'A Public Health Approach to the Problem of Obesity' in the chapter dealing with prevention, and to Tam Fry of the Child Growth Foundation for permission to use the BMI Charts which appear in Appendix 4 and for introducing me to the 'Cole Calculator'.

Mrs Jean Scott, Mrs Karen Mould, Miss Johanna-Maria Deahl and particularly Mrs Anna Sperring have been of immense help in preparing the manuscript and Marcela Holmes and Gina Almond of Blackwell Science have been unfailingly courteous and encouraging.

Introduction and overview

In 1976 a Department of Health and Social Security/Medical Research Council group concluded that

'We are unanimous in our belief that obesity is a hazard to health and a detriment to wellbeing. It is common enough to constitute one of the most important medical and public health problems of our time whether we judge importance by a shorter expectation of life, increased morbidity, or cost to the community in terms of both money and anxiety.' (James 1976)

Twenty-five years on from then, the position has, in fact, worsened.

Obesity is a major medical problem, yet it is trivialized in the media and marginalized by the Health Service. The World Health Organization (WHO), despite its historical focus on malnutrition and starvation, has for the first time recognized the problem of overnutrition. In 1998, the WHO said 'The epidemic projections for the next decade are so serious that public health action is urgently required' (WHO 1998), and again in 2000 (WHO 2000) it called for urgent action to combat the growing epidemic of obesity which now affects developing and industrialized countries alike.

The United Kingdom (UK) is currently experiencing an epidemic of overweight and obesity. Over 6 million people in the UK are obese. The prevalence of serious obesity doubled in Britain between 1980 and 1991 and is continuing to increase.

Over the past 20 years in all affluent nations there has been an explosion of overweight individuals who will increase the health care demands for diabetes, hypertension, heart disease, gall bladder disease, some forms of cancer and osteoarthritis over the coming decades (Bray 1999).

Even in the developing countries a pattern of rapidly escalating obesity and its comorbidities is becoming apparent in certain sections of society. Prentice (Prentice 2000) has cited the Gambia as an example, pointing out that rural poverty and malnutrition now vie with the diseases of urban prosperity—obesity and type 2 diabetes—for scarce health care resources. Current projections predict that the rise in obesity and type 2 diabetes in the developing world will outstrip that of the west; this adding another health burden to countries already beleaguered by famine and disease.

Obesity is the major nutritional disorder facing westernized civilizations and has become a major economic burden to most developed countries. It accounts for between 4% and 8% of total healthcare expenditure and is assuming increasing importance as a disease entity, with a massive impact on mortality, morbidity and the quality of life of those unfortunate enough to bear its consequences. Currently overweight and obesity may account for as much as 30% of coronary heart disease and 75% of new cases of type 2 diabetes (Jung 1997). However, coronary heart disease and type 2 diabetes are but two of the major conditions associated with obesity—other disabling conditions should not be ignored because obesity contributes to disorders of systems, e.g. cardiovascular and respiratory; to disorders of metabolism, e.g. insulin resistance and hyperlipidaemia; and to the development of site-specific cancers, e.g. colorectal, bilary system, or uterine, as well as cancers of the cervix and ovary.

The American Heart Association has recently upgraded obesity from a contributing risk factor to a major risk factor for coronary heart disease, thereby acknowledging that obesity is a lifelong disease that is becoming a dangerous epidemic with high rates of morbidity and mortality.

The fact is that in spite of our imperfect knowledge of all the factors that lead to obesity, people can be helped to lose weight and to maintain weight loss; but achieving this on a large scale will require fundamental changes in the way that society in general and health professionals in particular view the management of obesity. It is not simply a question of gluttony or sloth (Prentice & Jebb 1995).

Unfortunately many members of the public and, indeed, many health professionals often view obesity simply as a problem of eating too much and exercising too little, when in fact it is a complex, multifactorial disease of appetite regulation and energy metabolism that involves genetics, physiology, biochemistry and the neurosciences as well as environmental, psychological and cultural factors (Thomas 1995).

Obesity, of course, is not increasing because people are consciously trying to gain weight. In fact, millions of people in this country are dieting at any one time; they and many others are struggling to manage their weight to improve their appearance, feel better and become healthier. Obesity is a remarkable disease in terms of the discrimination its victims suffer and the efforts required by an individual for its successful management.

Obese people, like people with physical handicaps, wear their problem for all to see at all times; yet, unlike that group, they are held responsible for their condition (Wooley et al. 1979a, 1979b). Prejudice against fat people starts at school, affects their jobs and social opportunities and is so pervasive that it can colour the attitudes of professionals.

In the last few years there has been renewed interest in the use of drugs to aid the successful management of obesity, and attitudes have liberalized to the extent that there is growing acknowledgement that the treatment of obesity, like the treatment of hypertension, may have to be continued over long periods of time.

The goals of obesity treatment need to be refocused from weight loss alone to weight management, and success judged more on the effects on the overall health of individuals rather than on the achievement of ideal body weight. Because the increasing prevalence of overweight and obesity represents a most pervasive public health problem, it certainly deserves greater investment in both good quality research and service provision (Glennie *et al.* 1997).

Although obesity is a serious medical condition and is associated with a wide range of chronic and life-threatening conditions, 'although obese individuals suffer increased psycho-social problems and a reduced quality of life', and although the prevalence of obesity has enormous implications for the Health Service, it has not until quite recently attracted the scientific attention which its importance certainly deserves.

While the bad news is that the prevalence of obesity is rising, the good news that has emerged over the last few years is that relatively modest weight loss can have a major impact on reducing the risk factors for developing type 2 diabetes, cardiovascular disease and other obesity related conditions (Goldstein 1992).

Until quite recently the obese were urged to strive for the achievement of their ideal body weight, which required such massive changes in the eating habits and lifestyle of individuals that for the majority it was doomed to failure. One of the most important findings from recent research into obesity is the benefit to individuals of a 5–10% weight loss in improving their risk profile (James 1996). The fact that it is no longer necessary to strive for the well-nigh unachievable ideal body weight and that the benefits of the 5–10% reduction in weight are so considerable should motivate both doctors and patients to achieve the achievable. Effective weight management does not simply mean organizing a slimming process—it is a completely different concept geared to ensuring that the long-term health of the patient is the key concern.

While primary care is the obvious place for managing high risk individuals (see Chapter 7) there is also the need for a massive public health approach to reduce the prevalence of overweight and obesity in the population. Unfortunately a lack of success in treating obesity has led to a sense of frustration among general practitioners and practice nurses. To some extent this has been associated with the setting of unrealistic targets; for the severely obese person, achieving ideal body weight is just not a viable proposition.

Obesity is serious health problem which as much deserves a structured approach to its management as do hypertension and diabetes.

While diet and exercise will remain crucial to its effective management, drug therapy should certainly be considered in high-risk patients, as should the use of surgery for a limited group of people. No longer should obesity be regarded simply as a cosmetic issue, nor as a moral judgement on those who suffer from it.

References

Bennett, N., Dodd, T. & Flatley, J. (1996) *Health Survey for England 1993*. HMSO, London.

Bray, G.A. (1999) *Obesity: The Threat Ahead*. European Congress of Obesity, Germany, p. 42.

Glennie, A.M., O'Meara, S., Melville, A., Sheldon, T.A *et al*. (1997) The treatment and prevention of obesity: a systematic review of the literature. *International Journal of Obesity* **21**, 715–737.

Goldstein, D.J. (1992) Beneficial health effects of modest weight loss. *International Journal of Obesity* **16**, 397–415.

James, W.P.T. (1976) *Research on Obesity: a report of a DHSS/MRC Group*. HMSO, London.

James, W.P.T. (1996) The International Obesity Task Force; Obesity at the World Health Organisation. *Nutrition, Metabolism and Cardiovascular Disease Supplement* **6**, 12–13.

Jung, R.T. (1997) Obesity as a disease. *British Medical Bulletin* **53**, 307–321.

Prentice, A.M. (2000) Urban obesity in the Gambia. *Obesity in Practice* **2**, 2–5.

Prentice, A.M & Jebb, S.A. (1995) Obesity in Britain: Gluttony or Sloth? *British Medical Journal* **311**, 437–439.

Thomas, P.R. (ed.) (1995) *Weighing the Options*. National Academy Press, Washington.

Wooley, S.C., Wooley, O.W. & Dyrenforth, S.R. (1979a) Obesity and women II—A neglected feminist topic. *Women's Studies International Quarterly* **2**, 81–92.

Wooley, S.C., Wooley, O.W. & Dyrenforth, S.R. (1979b) Theoretical, practical and social issues in behavioural treatments of obesity. *Journal of Applied Behaviour Analysis* **12**, 3–25.

World Health Organization (1998) *Prevention and Management of the Global Epidemic of Obesity*. Report of the WHO consultation on obesity, Geneva 1997.WHO, Geneva.

World Health Organization (2000) *Preventing and Managing the Global Epidemic*. Report of the WHO Consultation. WHO Technical Report Series 894. Geneva, Switzerland.

2 Epidemiology

DEFINITION, CLASSIFICATION AND IDENTIFICATION

It has been traditional to define obesity in terms of a particular individual's body mass index (BMI). Although this can be criticized on the grounds that differences in weight between individuals are only partly due to variations in body fat, the fact remains that there is a very good correlation between BMI and the percentage of body fat in large populations.

$$\text{Body Mass Index} = \frac{\text{weight in kgs}}{(\text{Height in m})^2}$$

The World Health Organization and International Obesity Task Force definitions of obesity are shown in Fig. 2.1.

There are, however, drawbacks to using this measurement in clinical practice:

1 It usually requires recourse to tables.
2 Height must be measured accurately because errors are exaggerated by squaring.
3 More importantly it fails to distinguish general from truncal obesity and it is the latter which is related to the presence of a constellation of risk factors including insulin resistance, hyperinsulinaemia, decreased glucose tolerance, decreased HDL cholesterol, elevated LDL cholesterol and triglycerides, and hypertension—often known collectively as syndrome X, the metabolic syndrome, or Reaven's syndrome. It is today's people with syndrome X who will be tomorrow's victims of type 2 diabetes, coronary heart disease and other vascular disorders.

Fig 2.1 WHO and IOTF definitions of obesity for adults (men and women).

Normal BMI	18.5–24.9
Overweight BMI	
Pre-obese	25.0–29.9
Obesity Class I	30.0–34.9
Obesity Class II	35.0–39.9
Obesity Class III	More than 40

For busy clinicians, waist measurement is emerging as an alternative to calculating BMI (Han *et al.* 1995). Sex-specific waist measurement in relation to risk can be seen in Fig. 2.2.

The waist : hip ratio has been a traditional method of identifying people with prominent truncal obesity, but recent research has shown the value of using the waist circumference alone. This should be measured at half-way between the superior iliac crest and the ribcage in the mid-axilliary line. For busy primary care workers, waist measurement is a more practical tool than calculating BMI.

The above figures apply to people of Caucasian origin; for people of Asian origin there is a substantial risk for women above 80 cm and men above 88 cm waist circumference.

In fact, using BMI alone only has a positive predictive value of central obesity of 64% in men and 84% in women and will therefore miss a considerable number of people at high risk of developing type 2 diabetes and circulatory disorders. The circumference of the waist relates closely to BMI, is the dominant measurement in waist : hip ratio, and reflects the proportion of body fat located intra-abdominally as opposed to subcutaneously (Lean *et al.* 1995). The simplicity of waist measurement and its relationship to body weight, fat distribution and a clustering of cardiovascular risk factors, suggests that it could well have a place in primary care in identifying the 'at risk'.

IMPORTANCE OF FAT DISTRIBUTION

The distribution of excess adipose tissue is closely linked to the development of the major risk factors associated with obesity. Vague (Vague 1956) pointed out the strong association between android (upper-body or truncal) obesity and the development of type 2 diabetes mellitus. Truncal obesity, sometimes referred to as 'apple shaped', is significantly more strongly associated with the development of risk factors than gynoid (gluteo-femoral or 'pear shaped') obesity. Android obesity is now recognized as 'a feature of the syndrome of insulin resistance' (sometimes known as the metabolic syndrome, syndrome X or Reaven's syndrome), which includes compensatory hyperinsulinism, dyslipidaemia, hypertension, glucose intolerance, a pro-coagulant tendency

Fig 2.2 Sex-specific waist measurement related to risk.

	Increased risk	**Substantial risk**
Men	At or greater than 94 cm (approximately 37")	At or greater than 102 cm (approximately 40")
Women	At or greater than 80 cm (approximately 32")	At or greater than 88 cm (approximately 35")

and accelerated atheroma formation (Reaven 1988). This will be further discussed in Chapter 5.

The importance of waist measurement over BMI is that it does recognize the importance of intra-abdominal fat accumulation and its greater relevance to accompanying risk factors. Figure 2.3 shows the relationship between waist measurement and odds ratio for risk factors.

Intra-abdominal fat accumulation is often indicative of a constellation of risk factors which include insulin resistance and hyperinsulinaemia, hypertension, dyslipidaemia (raised total cholesterol), LDL cholesterol and triglycerides and lowered HDL cholesterol which markedly increase an individual's risk of developing coronary heart disease.

PREVALENCE

The prevalence of obesity in a population refers to the percentage of people in that population with excess storage of body fat and it has increased by about 10–40% in most developed countries in the past decade. During this period the prevalence in the UK has doubled (Fig. 2.4).

In 1996 16% of men and 18% of women were obese and a further 45% of men and 34% of women were overweight. One percent of the population was categorized as severely obese. The Health of the Nation report one year on pointed out that over half of the adult male population and just under half of the adult female population were overweight to a clinically undesirable degree. Men tend to predominate in the category BMI 25–30, whereas there are more women than men who are obese (BMI 30–40) or severely obese (BMI >40). About a quarter of

Fig 2.3 Relationship between waist measurement and odds ratio for risk factors.

| | Men | | Women | |
	At Risk	High Risk	At Risk	High Risk
Waist measurement (cm)	94–102	>102	80–88	>88
Odds ratio for risk factors	2.2 (1.8–2.8)	4.6 (3.5–6.0)	0.6 (1.3–2.1)	2.6 (2.0–3.2)

Risk factors: ≥ 6.5mmol/l cholesterol
≤ 0.9mmol/l HDL cholesterol
≥ 160 or > 95mmHg systolic and diastolic BP

From Han *et al*.1995.

all adults are estimated to be dieting at any one time. Health of the Nation 1992 targeted a reduction in the proportion of obese people (BMI >30) to not more than 6% of men and 8% of women by the year 2005. The growing world epidemic of obesity is shown graphically in Fig. 2.5.

COMORBID CONDITIONS

Obesity and overweight are associated with an increased risk of developing type 2 diabetes, hypertension, coronary heart disease, stroke, and gall bladder disease, as well as certain cancers (Jung 1997). In addition, obese people are often discriminated against socially and tend to have low self-esteem. In males the greatest correlation is with colorectal cancer, whereas in females it is with endometrial cancer, followed by cancer of the gall bladder and biliary tract. Also, in females, excessive obesity is associated with an increased risk of breast, cervical and ovarian cancers (Lew & Garfinkel 1987).

In addition, obesity and overweight contribute to the development of osteoarthritis, breathlessness, dyspepsia, sleep apnoea and venous thromboembolism; they make pregnancy, anaesthesia and surgery more hazardous; and they contribute to psychological distress and low self-esteem (*Drug & Therapeutics Bulletin* 1998).

Fig 2.4 Recent trends in the prevalence of obesity.

Country definition	Obesity	Year	Ages	Men (%)	Women (%)
ENGLAND	30kg/m²	1980	16–64	6	8
		1986–87		7	12
		1991		13	15
		1993		13	16
USA	30kg/m²	1960	20–74	10.0	15.0
		1973		11.6	16.1
		1978		12.0	14.8
		1991		19.7	24.7
GERMANY	30kg/m²	1985	25–69	15.1	16.5
		1988		14.7	17.2
		1990		17.2	19.3

Fig 2.5 The growing epidemic of obesity.

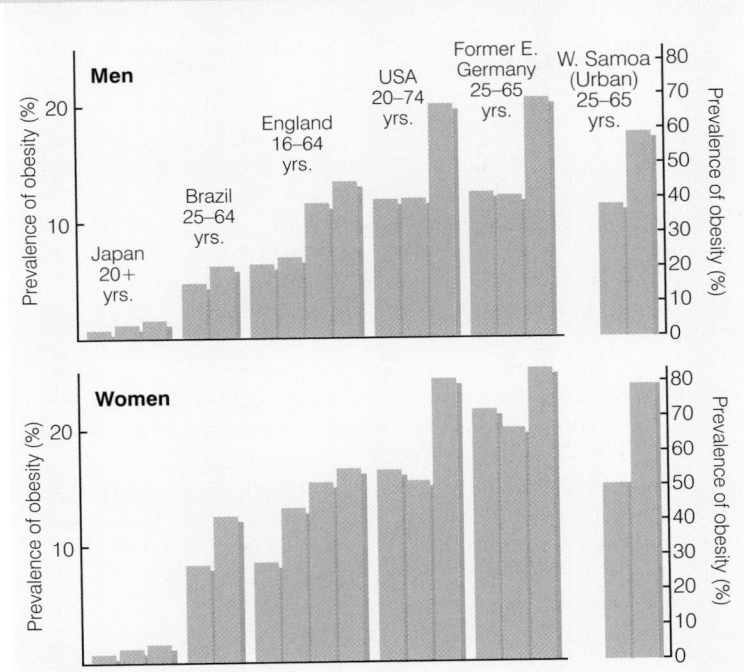

References

Anon. (1998) Why and how should adults lose weight. *Drug and Therapuetics Bulletin* **36** (12), 89–92.

Han, T.S., Van Leer, E.M., Seidell, J.C. *et al.* (1995) Waist circumference action levels in the identification of cardiovascular risk factors–prevalence study in a random sample. *British Medical Journal* **311**, 1401–1405.

Jung, R.T. (1997) Obesity as a disease. *British Medical Bulletin* **53**, 307–321.

Lew, E.A. & Garfinkel, D. (1987) Variation in mortality by weight among 750,000 men and women. *Journal of Chronic Diseases* **32**, 563–576.

Reaven, G.M. (1988) Role of insulin resistance in human disease. *Diabetes* **37**, 1595–1607.

Vague, J. (1956) The degree of masculine differentiation of obesities; the factor determining predisposition to diabetes, atherosclerosis, gout and uric calculus disease. *American Journal of Clinical Nutrition* **4**, 20–34.

3 Causes of obesity

HEREDITY

A review of studies involving more than 10 000 individuals from biological and adoptive relationships. It determined the correlation of BMI for monozygotic and dizygotic twins and for the biological parent–offspring and adoptive–relative pairs. It found a weighted mean BMI correlation of 0.74 for monozygotic twins and 0.32 for dizygotic twin pairs. This corresponds to an estimated hereditibility of between 50% and 90%.

In addition the correlations for biological parent–offspring pairs and adoptive pairs were 0.19 and 0.06, respectively. This indicates a relatively minor role for the cultural transmission of obesity.

GENETIC AND FAMILIAL

Studies in Denmark (Stunkard *et al.* 1986; Sorensen *et al.* 1989) have given substance to there being a genetic component to obesity; they studied adoptees and twins. Studies of adoptees showed great correlation between their weight and that of their biological, but not their adopted, parents and siblings. Twin studies showed great intrapair correlation coefficients regardless of whether they were reared together or apart. The researchers have postulated that genetic influences on BMI could account for up to 70% of variants. However, this may well be an exaggerated claim since in epidemiological terms the escalating rates of obesity, which affect large sections of the population, have occurred in a relatively constant gene pool. This suggests that the primary causes lie in environmental and behavioural change (Prentice & Jebb 1995). Children of families where one or both parents are obese are certainly at increased risk of becoming obese themselves (Guillaume *et al.* 1993).

DEMOGRAPHIC FACTORS

Increasing obesity is associated with:
- Increasing age—at least, up to 50–60 years of age in men and women.
- Gender—women generally have a higher prevalence of obesity, especially when over 50 years of age.
- Ethnicity—there are large and often unexplained variations between ethnic groups.

SOCIO-CULTURAL FACTORS

Risk of obesity is associated with social class (Kahn *et al.* 1991). In England 1994 age standardized prevalence of obesity in women was 12% and 14% in Classes 1 and 2, compared with 22% and 21% in Social Classes 4 and 5. For men the variations are less: prevalence is 10% in Social Class 1, compared with 14% and 13% in Social Classes 4 and 5.

Educational status is also an influence. Women with no educational qualifications show a mean BMI of $26.7 \, \text{kg/m}^2$ compared with $24.6 \, \text{kg/m}^2$ in those educated to A Level and above (Colhoun & Prescott-Clarke 1996).

Being married is often associated with an increased chance of becoming obese.

BIOLOGICAL FACTORS

While it has been claimed that BMI increases with increasing parity, recent evidence suggests that this contribution is likely to be small—less than 1 kg per pregnancy (Williamson *et al.* 1994).

BEHAVIOURAL CHANGE FACTORS

Physical inactivity

There are a number of behavioural influences of which probably decreasing physical activity is of major importance and likely to be the main factor behind age-related weight gain (Prentice & Jebb 1995). As the nation's epidemic of obesity has occurred during decades of reducing food intake, the implication must be that levels of energy expenditure decline even more rapidly. Support for this view comes from the following evidence.

Mechanisms for regulating body weight were evolved historically under conditions of high physical activity. The increasing affluence of the postwar years has been matched by the adoption of increasingly sedentary lifestyles: only 20% of men and 10% of women are currently employed in physically active occupations (Allied Dunbar 1992). Physically active leisure pursuits have been replaced by inactive pastimes. The average person now watches television 26 h a week compared with 13 h in the 1960s. The Health Survey for England (Colhoun & Prescott-Clarke 1996) and the Allied Dunbar National Fitness Survey revealed that in the previous month:

- 30–35% of men had taken fewer than four 20-minute periods of moderate activity;

- 80% of men had not walked continuously for two miles;
- only 20–30% of men had participated in vigorous activity of any type.

In a Finnish study (Rissanen *et al.* 1991) of 1200 adults over a 5-year period it was concluded that physical inactivity was more important than diet as a cause of obesity (See Fig. 3.1).

English activity patterns have probably fallen by an average of 800 kcal/day over the past 20 years (James 1995) while food intake has fallen by about 750 kcal/day. The result is a small but sustained imbalance between intake and output which has to be a major contributory factor in the development of the current epidemic of obesity.

Declining physical activity has been matched by the adoption of increasingly sedentary lifestyles. The eating of high-fat diets and small, frequent snacks contributes to obesity because they reduce the conscious recognition that food is being eaten and bypass feelings of satiety. In fact, 1 g of fat provides more than twice as many calories as the same quantity of carbohydrate or protein. High-fat diets, which are often palatable without inducing feelings of satiety, are certainly contributory. Fat, unlike protein or carbohydrate, induces only a small rise in metabolic rate.

'Faced by a life circumstance that discourages routine physical effort and activity and that offers a surfeit of highly palatable high energy and high fat foods in bewildering variety, weight gain is an understandable consequence' (Hill & Rogers 1998).

All of the above information has important messages for the design of weight-loss and weight-maintenance programmes.

Dietary intake

During the last 50 years there has been a marked increase in the fat content of the British diet (MAFF 1994) and there is evidence that high fat consumption undermines the mechanisms regulating energy balance. The eating of high-fat diets and small, frequent snacks contribute to obesity because they reduce the conscious recognition that food is being eaten and bypass feelings of satiety. Although dietary studies suggest an association between obesity and high fat consumption, they suffer from the well known unreliability of the recording of food intake. However, a study of 11 600 Scottish men and women (Bolton-Smith & Woodward

Fig 3.1 Physical inactivity – a dominant factor in causing obesity.

- Increasing use of motorized transport
- Energy sparing domestic devices
- Lifts and escalators
- Obsessive television watching
- Video games
- Overuse of central heating

1994) related the prevalence of obesity to the subjects' intakes of sugars and fat. This study showed quite clearly that the groups consuming the highest proportion of their energy from carbohydrate were much less likely to be obese compared with low sugar, high fat consumers. Laboratory studies lend support to these findings:

- The observation that the consumption of food is associated with an increase in energy expenditure and oxygen consumption was made by Lavoisier over 200 years ago. This effect is now termed the 'thermic effect of food' (or 'dietary-induced thermogenesis').
- There is now experimental evidence to show that the thermic effect of carbohydrate vastly exceeds the thermic effect of fat.
- Mechanisms for regulating body weight function more effectively on a high carbohydrate, low-fat diet than on a high-fat, low-carbohydrate diet.
- Carbohydrate balance is accurately regulated by increases in oxidation which are regulated by the autonomic nervous system and help to compensate for excess energy intake.
- In humans, isotope studies have shown *de novo* fat synthesis from carbohydrate is a minor process.
- Fat is less satiating.

Energy expenditure

Carbohydrate and fat are, under normal conditions, the main sources of energy for man. Carbohydrate is stored as glycogen in the liver and muscle, while fat is stored as triglyceride in adipose tissue.

There is a much closer correlation between energy intake and expenditure with carbohydrate than there is with fat.

Total energy expenditure: Resting energy expenditure and unrestricted physical exercise (Schoeller 1990).

- Basal Metabolic Rate 70%.
- Thermic Effect of Food 10%.
- Spontaneous Physical Activity 20%.

The above percentages are averages—there are wide personal variations between individuals (Flatt 1998).

Basal metabolic rate (BMR) is determined by the free fat mass, the total body mass, age and gender. Thermogenesis (thermic effect of food) is greater after carbohydrate intake than it is after fat intake. Spontaneous physical activity (fidgeting movements) varies considerably between individuals.

Factors related to energy expenditure which could contribute to obesity are therefore:

- Low BMR;
- Defects in the thermogenic effect of food;
- Low levels of spontaneous physical activity.

DYNAMICS OF WEIGHT GAIN

- When energy intake equals energy expenditure, body weight is constant.
- When intake begins to exceed expenditure even by relatively small amounts, the slide down the slippery slope towards being overweight and, if unchecked, towards obesity, has begun (See Fig. 3.2).
- After a period of time a new equilibrium is reached and weight tends to plateau.

Metabolic predictors of weight gain

Studies on Pima Indians, a race which is exceptionally prone to obesity, suggest that a low resting BMR and low levels of spontaneous physical activity induce a future tendency to obesity (Ravussin *et al.* 1988).

The fact that there is also a familial tendency towards a low BMR suggests that genetic influences could also play a part.

Similar familial tendencies towards low levels of spontaneous physical activity have also been demonstrated—again suggesting that genetic influences could be relevant. Spontaneous physical activity is strongly influenced by the sympathetic nervous system.

SYMPATHO—ADRENAL SYSTEM AND OBESITY

The sympathetic nervous system (SNS) and the adrenal medulla together make up the sympatho-adrenal system, which has a major role in maintaining homeostasis.

Its effects are mediated:
- Directly by the sympathetic nerves which supply most parts of the body;
- Indirectly by catecholamines, adrenaline and noradrenaline released from the adrenal medulla. These enter the blood stream and act as hormones at target sites around the body.

The SNS can influence the development of obesity by influencing:
- Food intake;
- Energy expenditure;
- Resting BMR;
- Fat balance.

Fig 3.2 Energy balance.

A positive energy balance of 2 kcal/day could increase body weight by about 1kg in 10 years

Seidall J.C., Flegal K.M. 1997

Food intake

A high SNS drive inhibits food intake (Bray *et al*. 1989; Bray 1991).

Studies have shown a strong correlation between postprandial suppression of hunger and noradrenaline response—as an indicator of SNS activity.

Energy expenditure

In summary, increased SNS actively increases energy expenditure by its action through B1 and B2 adrenergenic receptors and by increasing the thermogenic effect of food.

Resting BMR

People with low SNS activity have a lower BMR which could predispose them to obesity, and possibly a higher food intake (see above).

Fat balance

Beta-adrenergic blockade in humans leads to a moderate increase in carbohydrate and protein oxidation but a substantial decrease in fat oxidation, which suggests that of all the macronutrients—carbohydrate, fat and protein—the oxidation of fat is most dependent on sympathetic stimulation.

Clearly then, any lack of this stimulation will increase the likelihood of obesity.

Alcohol consumption

Moderate or heavy alcohol consumption can be associated with a high BMI (Prentice 1995).

Smoking cessation

Smoking cessation is an important risk factor for weight gain in either sex (Flagal *et al*. 1995). In one study, weight gain as a result of smoking cessation averaged 2.8 kg in males and 3.8 kg in females (Williamson *et al*. 1991). The weight gain results from a decrease in energy expenditure. Each cigarette utilizes 8 kcal by stimulation of the SNS. Smoking also curbs the appetite, which tends to increase after stopping.

Age

The risk of obesity for men increases during their late 30s. Women, however, face an increased risk at several stages in their lives: for example after marriage, during pregnancy, during the menopause and at retirement (Sorensen in Department of Health 1995).

Ethnicity

The risk of obesity may vary between different ethnic groups. Asian people are at greater risk of developing obesity than Afro-Caribbean and Caucasian people (NHS 1996). Many Asian people have a central body fat distribution and its related comorbidities even when their BMI is not in the obese range.

South Asian people are particularly at risk of developing abdominal obesity. There is also an increased prevalence of insulin resistance in this group.

Drugs

Certain drugs can increase appetite and promote weight gain. The commonest are anabolic agents, steroids, some oral contraceptives, sulphonylureas, tricyclic antidepressants, lithium, and some benzodiazepines.

Endocrine and hypothalamic causes

A number of endocrine and hypothalamic disorders contribute to the development of obesity and are listed in Fig. 3.3.

However, these make only a minor contribution to the current epidemic of obesity and therefore are not discussed in any detail. Readers wishing to know more about them are recommended to consult a textbook on endocrinology.

CONCLUSION

It is hoped that the foregoing will suggest to the reader that energy balance and the development of obesity are not much more complicated than a simple measure of calories in and calories out.

The development of obesity involves complex interactions between gender and environmental influences and at least some of these are

Fig 3.3 Endocrine causes of obesity.

Decreased energy expenditure
Hypothyroidism

Increased energy intake
Cushing's disease
Hypogonadism in men
Insulinoma
Growth hormone deficiency

The Stein–Leventhal Syndrome (polycystic ovary) also contributes to obesity but the exact mechanism remains to be elucidated. It could be due to altered ovarian function or hypersensitivity of the hypothalamic–pituitary–adrenal axis

Hypothalamic causes
Tumours
Damage by irradiation or infection
Prader–Willi syndrome – thought to be caused by a hypothalamic disorder

mediated via hormones and the autonomic nervous system— largely beyond conscious influence. Therefore it is little wonder that tackling the problems of obesity is so challenging. Perhaps the first key change is for health workers to appreciate the complexity of the problem—that it is not a simple matter of 'gluttony or sloth'—and begin to treat obese people with the respect and compassion that the complexity of their condition deserves.

The influence of the SNS on both energy intake and expenditure has very important implications for the development of drug treatments and the prevention and management of obesity.

References

Allied Dunbar (1992) *National Fitness Survey: a report on activity patterns and fitness levels*. Sports Council and Health Education Authority, London.

Bolton-Smith, C. & Woodward, M. (1994) Dietary composition and fat to sugar ratios in relation to obesity. *International Journal of Obesity* **18**, 820–828.

Bray, G.A. (1991) Reciprocal relation between the sympathetic nervous system and food intake. *Brain Research Bulletin* **27**, 517–520,

Bray, G.A., York, D.A. & Fisher, J.S. (1989) Experimental Obesity: a homeostasis failure due to defective nutrient stimulation of the sympathetic nervous system. *Vitamins Hormones* **45**, 1–125.

Colhoun, H. & Prescott-Clarke, P., eds. (1996) *Health survey for England 1994: a survey carried out on behalf of the Department of Health,* vol. 1. HMSO, London, p. 1.449.

Department of Health (1995) *Obesity: Reversing the Increasing Problem of Obesity in England.* A report from the Nutritional and Physical Activity Task Forces.

Flagal, K.M., Troiano, R.P., Pamuck, E.R. *et al.* (1995) The influence of smoking cessation on the prevalence of over weight in the United States. *New England Journal of Medicine* **333**, 1165–1170.

Flatt, J.P. (1998) Importance of nutrient balance in body weight regulation. *Diabetes Metabolism Review* **18**, 820–828

Guillaume, M., Lapidus, L., Beckers, F. *et al.*(1993) Prevalence of obesity in Belgian Luxembourg. *International Journal of Obesity* **17**, (suppl. 2), 36.

Hill, A.J. & Rogers, P.G. (1998) Food intake and eating behaviour. In: *Clinical Obesity* (eds P. G. Kopelman & M. J. Stock), pp. 86–111. Blackwell Science, Oxford.

James, W.P.T. (1995) A Public Health Approach to the problem of obesity. *International Journal of Obesity* **19** (Suppl. 3), 37–45.

Kahn, H.S., Williamson, D.F. & Stevens, J.A. (1991) Race and weight change in US women; the role of socio-economic and marital status. *American Journal of Public Health* **83**, 319–332.

Lew, E.A. & Garfinkel, D. (1987) Variation in mortality by weight among 750,000 men and women. *Journal of Chronic Diseases* **32**, 563–576.

MAFF (1994) *Household Food Consumption and Expenditure.* HMSO, London, 1940–94.

NHS CRD (1996) *Ethnicity and Health: reviews of literature and guidance for purchasers in the areas of CVD, mental health and haemoglobinopathy.* University of York, York, pp. 46–47.

Prentice, A.M. (1995) Alcohol and Obesity. *International Journal of Obesity* **19** (Suppl. 5), S44–S50.

Prentice, A.M. & Jebb, S.A. (1995) Obesity in Britain. gluttony or sloth? *British Medical Journal* **311**, 437–439.

Ravussin, E., Lillioja, S., Knowler, W.C. *et al*. (1988) Reduced rate of energy expenditure as a risk factor for body weight gain. *New England Journal of Medicine* **318**, 467–472.

Rissanen, A.M., Heliovaara, M., Knekt, P. *et al*. (1991) Determinants of weight gain and overweight in adult Finns. *European Journal of Clinical Nutrition* **45**, 419–430.

Schoeller, D.A. (1990) How accurate is self reported energy intake? *Nutrition Review* **48**, 373–379.

Sorensen, T.I., Price, R.A., Stunkard, A.J. *et al*. (1989) Genetics of obesity in adult adoptees and their biological siblings. *British Medical Journal* **298**, 87–90.

Stunkard, A.J., Sorensen, T.I., Hanis, C. *et al*. (1986) An adoption study of human obesity. *New England Journal of Medicine* **314**, 193–19813.

Williamson, D.F., Madans, J., Anda, R.F. *et al*. (1991) Smoking cessation and severity of weight gain in a national cohort. *New England Journal of Medicine* **324**, 739–745.

Williamson, D.F., Madans, J., Pamuk, E. *et al*. (1994) A prospective study of childbearing and 10 year weight gain in US white women 25–40 years age. *International Journal of Obesity* **18**, 561–569.

4 The autocrine, paracrine and endocrine functions of adipose tissue

COMPOSITION OF ADIPOSE TISSUE

Adipose tissue is a type of loose connective tissue made up of adipocytes surrounded by a matrix of collagen fibres, blood vessels, fibroblasts and immune cells. In the mesentery and subcutaneous tissues it is organized into large lobular structures. There are basically two types of adipose tissue: white and brown, of which white predominates in humans.

Brown fat only makes up a small percentage of total body fat; it is more abundant in infants but is present in adults as well. It is mainly located between the scapulas, at the nape of the neck and along the blood vessels in the thorax and abdomen. In brown fat depots the fat cells as well as the blood vessels have an extensive sympathetic innervation, which is in contrast to white fat depots in which there may be innervation of some fat cells but the principal sympathetic innervation is on blood vessels.

This extensive sympathetic innervation is responsible for activating dietary induced thermogenesis which in turn plays a part in energy regulation. Reduced sympathetic activation of brown adipose tissue is a feature of most models of obesity (Stock 1998).

White adipocytes have only a single large droplet of white fat, whereas brown fat cells contain several small droplets of fat (Gannong 1999).

Cellular lipids

The lipids in cells are of two main types: (i) structural lipids, which are an inherent part of the membranes and other parts of cells; and (ii) neutral fat, which is stored in the adipocytes of the fat depots. While neutral fat is mobilized during starvation, structural lipid is preserved. In the non-obese individual, fat depots make up about 15% of body weight in men and 21% in women. *Adipose tissue is not an inert mass but is actively involved in metabolism and energy homeostasis as well as having endocrine and paracrine functions.* In addition it influences autonomic and immune function (Flier & Spiegelman 1996; Mohammed-Ali *et al.* 1998).

INTERCELLULAR COMMUNICATION

This can occur by the following methods:
1   Neural communication, in which neurotransmitters are released at synaptic junctions.
2   Endocrine communication, in which hormones and growth factors reach cells via the blood stream.
3   Paracrine communication, in which the products of cells diffuse into the extracellular fluid to reach other cells.
4   Autocrine communication, in which cells secrete chemical messengers that bind to receptors on the same cell (Gannong 1999).

SECRETORY ROLE OF ADIPOSE TISSUE

Adipocytes, stroma cells and macrophages secrete a range of substances with autocrine, paracrine and endocrine functions (Fig. 4.1).

The roles of some of these substances will now be briefly outlined, beginning with leptin which is emerging as a hormone of considerable importance, some even comparing its importance to that of insulin.

Fig 4.1 Secretory role of adipose tissue.

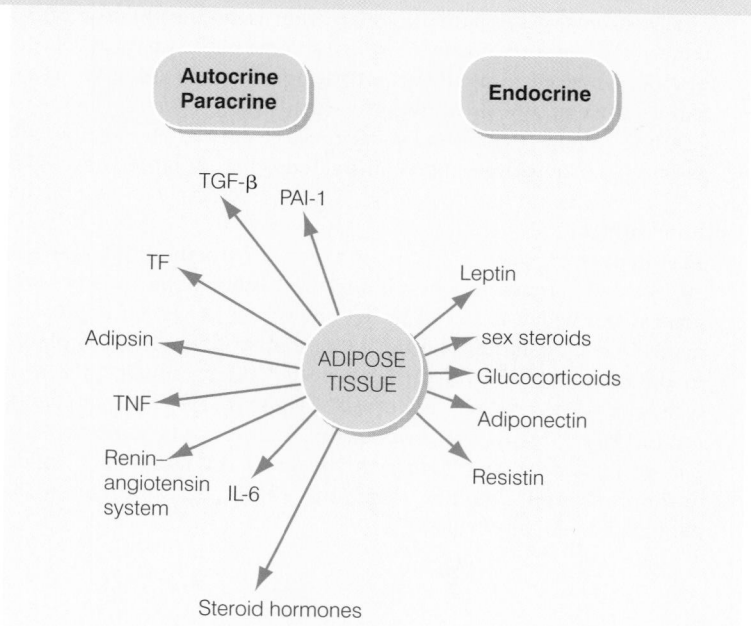

Leptin

Leptin was discovered in 1994 and is secreted mainly by adipose tissue, although low levels have been detected in the placenta, skeletal muscle, gastric and mammary epithelia, and brain (Freidman & Halaas 1998).

Circulating levels of leptin are related to body stores of energy and energy balance. They are high in obese individuals and low in lean people. Females tend to have higher leptin levels than males, probably as a result of an inhibitory effect by androgens.

Synthesis of leptin is higher in subcutaneous than visceral fat.

Deficiency of leptin results in hyperphagia, decreased energy expenditure and morbid obesity (however, in terms of human obesity leptin deficiency is rare).

Injection of leptin into the brain reduces food intake and reduces energy storage as fat. These findings led to the concept of leptin as an anti-obesity hormone. However, the high levels of leptin found in obese people clearly do not prevent its development. Also, clinical trials of injected leptin have yielded disappointing results. This has led to the development of the concept of leptin resistance (compare with insulin resistance).

It has been found that the CSF levels of leptin are considerably lower than serum levels in obese people (Schwartz *et al.* 2000). Thus failure to cross the blood–brain barrier could be a contributory factor to leptin resistance.

Leptin exerts its effect on the hypothalamus via a signalling system involving neuropeptide Y (NPY) and agouti-related protein (AGRP) which stimulate food intake, and melanocyte-stimulating hormone (MSH) and cocaine- and amphetamine-related transcript which reduce food intake. Thus an imbalance or failure of the signalling system could also be contributory to leptin resistance.

It does seem that leptin signals to the brain information about the size of the body's energy stores and the switch between the fed and fasted states (Flier 1998). Whilst trials of leptin have so far yielded disappointing results, knowledge about its signalling system has stimulated research into manipulating this for therapeutic purposes.

It could be that the future of leptin treatment could be more to do with maintaining than achieving weight loss.

Leptin has a range of other functions. Deficiency of leptin is associated with a failure of pubertal maturation. It also influences the immune system, being a potent mediator of immune suppresion during fasting (Lord *et al.* 1998).

Leptin also acts on the endocrine system, including the hypothalamo–pituitary axis, and influences the production of growth hormone and prolactin. It also activates the SNS and is involved in blood pressure regulation, brain and bone development, haematopoiesis, and wound healing (Ahima & Flier 2000).

An alternative hypothesis on the role of leptin is that of controlling the deposition of fat, preventing its harmful accumulation in tissues such as the heart, liver, and kidneys.

Interleukin 6 (IL-6)

IL-6 inhibits the lipoprotein lipase activity and increases aromotase activity. In addition it increases the production of free fatty acids and cholesterol by the liver. Levels of IL-6 rise with increasing BMI, especially if this is associated with abdominal obesity. It stimulates hepatic production of C reactive protein.

Tumour necrosis factor α

Tumour necrosis factor (TNF) has been suggested as a possible mediator of insulin resistance in obesity (Ahima & Flier 2000).

Renin–angiotensin system

The complete system is secreted by adipocytes. Levels are decreased by fasting and increased by re-feeding.

Angiotensin II, in addition to its role in regulating blood pressure, also increases the secretion of aromatase which in turn favours the conversion of androgens to oestrogens. It could contribute to the relationship between obesity, hypertension, and increased cardiovascular risk, and to the increased risk of breast and endometrial cancer in postmenopausal women.

Plasminogen activator inhibitor (PAI-1)

Plasmin (fibrinolysin) is the active component of the plasminogen (fibrinolysin) system. This enzyme lyses fibrinogen with the production of fibrinogen degradation products that inhibit thrombin. Plasmin is formed from its precursor plasminogen, a process which is prejudiced by plasminogen activator inhibitor (PAI-1) (Gannong 1999).

High levels of PAI-1 have been detected following myocardial infarction (Shimomura *et al.* 1996). While the liver is the main source of PAI-1 production, significant amounts are synthesized by adipose tissue and levels increase in direct proportion to visceral obesity. This could be another link between obesity and cardiovascular risk.

Adipsin (complement D)

This is a factor in stimulating the synthesis and storage of triglycerides; levels increase in response to human obesity and to feeding (Ahima & Flier 2000).

Adiponectin

This is secreted exclusively by adipocytes; levels are decreased in obesity, type 2 diabetes and coronary heart disease. It inhibits vascular smooth-muscle proliferation and expression of various adhesion molecules. The lower levels found in obesity could be contributory to the increased risk of CHD (Ahima & Flier 2000).

Steroid hormones

Adipose tissue has the ability to metabolize glucorcorticoids and sex steroid hormones (Sliteri 1987).

Oestrogens stimulate adipogenesis in the breast and subcutaneous tissue and androgens promote central obesity. Thus they play an important role in determining fat distribution and could influence the development of insulin resistance, type 2 diabetes and increased risk of CHD.

Resistin

The discovery of this hormone was first reported in *Nature* in January 2001 (Steppan *et al.* 2001).

The molecular links between obesity and type 2 diabetes have been elusive, yet the links are strong as 80% of people with type 2 diabetes are obese.

One of the fundamental defects in type 2 diabetes is insulin resistance.

The increased storage of triglycerides in adipose tissue in obesity is a factor in causing this tissue to be insulin resistant; but how is this linked to insulin resistance in the liver, skeletal muscle and other body tissues? For some time it has been believed that the non-esterified fatty acids secreted by adipocytes play a part: they probably do so, by substrate competition in skeletal muscle.

Tumour necrosis factor secreted by adipocytes could also be a factor in insulin resistance.

Now Steppan and colleagues, utilizing the fact that thiazolidinidiones reverse insulin resistance, have discovered another hormone that they have named resistin.

By treating a differentiated adipocyte cell line with thiazolidinidiones, they have identified a new messenger which is apparently only expressed by adipocytes. The evidence that resistin is involved in insulin resistance is provocative but as yet only circumstantial (Flier 2001).

The experiments by Steppan and colleagues show that resistin suppresses insulin's ability to stimulate the uptake of glucose by adipocytes. Whether it is able to do this in liver, muscle and other tissue awaits elucidation.

References

Ahima, R.S. *et al.* (1996) Role of leptin in the neuroendocrine response to fasting. *Nature* **382**, 250–252.

Ahima, R.S. & Flier, J.S. (2000) Adipose tissue as an endocrine organ. *Trends in Endocrinology and Metabolism* **11** (8), 327–332.

Flier, J.S. (1998) Clinical Review 94, What's in a name? In search of leptin's physiologic role. *Journal of Clinical Endocrine and Metabolism* **83**, 1407–1413.

Flier, J.S. (2001) The missing link with obesity? *Nature* **409**, 292–293.

Flier, J.S. & Spiegelman, B.M. (1996) Adipogenesis and obesity: rounding out the big picture. *Cell* **87**, 377–389.

Friedman, J.M. & Halaas, J.L. (1998) Leptin and the regulation of body weight in mammals. *Nature* **395**, 763–770.

Gannong, W. (1999) *Review of Medical Physiology*, 19th edn. Appleton & Lange, p. 519.

Lord, G.M. *et al.* (1998) Leptin modulates the T cell immune response and reverses starvation induced immunosuppresion. *Nature* **294**, 897–891.

Mohammed-Ali, V. *et al.* (1998) Adipose tissue as an endocrine and paracrine organ. *International Journal of Obesity* **22**, 1145–1158.

Schwartz, M.W., Woods, S.C., Ponte Jr, D. *et al.* (2000) Central nervous system control of food intake. *Nature* **404**, 661–671.

Shimomura, I., Funahashi, T., Takahashi, M. *et al.* (1996) Enhanced expression of PAI-I in visceral fat: possible contributor to vascular disease in obesity. *Nature Medicine* **2**, 800–803.

Sliteri, P.K. (1987) Adipose tissue as a source of hormones. *American Journal of Clinical Nutrition* **5** (Suppl.) (297–282), 13.

Steppan, C.M., Bailey, S.T., Bhat, S. *et al.* (2001) The hormone resistin links obesity to diabetes. *Nature* **409**, 307–312.

Stock, M.J. (1998) Energy balance and animal models of obesity. In: *Clinical Obesity* (eds P. G. Kopelmann & M. J. Stock), pp. 50–72. Blackwell Science, Oxford.

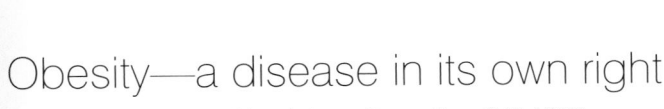

5 Obesity—a disease in its own right!

Obesity is not just a health risk but a disease (Jung R.T. 1997)

INTRODUCTION

The contribution of obesity to the development of some of the major chronic diseases affecting western civilization is quite staggering. For instance, above a BMI of 35 kg/m^2, women have a 93-fold increase in their risk of developing diabetes mellitus, and men a 42-fold increase.

It is paradoxical that although the medical profession is willing to recognize and treat the complications of obesity, such as type 2 diabetes, coronary heart disease and hypertension, it has been much less willing to accord obesity the status of a disease in its own right and devote to it the time and attention that it deserves (Fig. 5.1). Given the now proven links with mortality and morbidity, surely the time has come for a different approach—an approach that recognizes the disease of obesity and accords it the degree of attention that is seen as being appropriate for any major chronic condition that threatens the lifespan and the quality of life of those who experience it.

OBESITY AND MORTALITY

The Nurses' Health Study (Manson *et al*. 1995) has yielded valuable information about the link between overall mortality and morbidity from specific diseases in a cohort of 115 195 women in the USA who were between 35 and 55 years of age when enrolled into the study in 1976. In the 16-year follow-up period there were 4726 deaths, of which:

- 881 were due to cardiovascular disease;

Fig 5.1 Obesity, a disease in its own right because ......

- It causes extensive human suffering
- It has a major genetic component which interacts with environmental factors
- It has a massive financial cost to society
- It deserves a plan of management equal to those related to diabetes, asthma and hypertension
- If effectively managed it could bring significant benefits to the quality and quantity of human life.

- 2586 were due to cancer;
- 1259 were from other causes.
  In non-smokers the relative risk of death related to body weight was:
- 1.3 for BMI 25–26.9.
- 1.6 for BMI 27–28.9.
- 2.1 for BMI 29–31.

It was concluded that 53% of all deaths in women with BMI ≥29 were directly related to their obesity. Lean women (BMI <19), has the lowest mortality rates after correction for smoking and subclinical disease.

In a study of 750 000 men and women (Lew & Garfinkel 1979), relative mortality was highest for diabetes mellitus, followed by digestive diseases including cancer. Mortality from cancer was highest for colorectal cancer in males (1.73 in males, 1.22 in females), whereas in females it was highest for endometrial cancer, followed by cancer of the biliary tract. Substantial obesity was also associated with an increased risk of cancer of the cervix, breast and ovary (Fig. 5.2).

OBESITY AND MORBIDITY

In addition to having a marked effect on mortality, obesity also has a major impact on morbidity. Some of these effects are organ specific, e.g. breast (increased risk of cancer), skin (increased risk of fungal infection); others relate to systems, e.g. cardiovascular (increased risk of coronary heart disease and stroke); while others relate to functions, e.g. metabolism (increased risk of type 2 diabetes), and pregnancy (increased risk of obstetric complications). All these effects are summarized in Fig. 5.3.

Fig 5.2 Mortality risks in obesity.

	Males	Females
Diabetes	5.19	7.90
Digestive diseases	3.99	2.29
Coronary heart disease	1.85	2.07
Cerebro vascular disease	2.27	1.52
Cancer: all sites	1.33	1.55
Cancer: colorectal	1.73	
Cancer: prostate	1.29	
Cancer: gallbladder/biliary		3.58
Cancer: endometrium		5.42
Cancer: cervix		2.39
Cancer; ovary		1.63

OBESITY AND DIABETES

Type 2 diabetes is the most important medical consequence of obesity and becomes progressively commoner in populations with higher prevalences of obesity. It accounts for about 80–85% of the estimated 110 million people with diabetes worldwide—a number which is likely to increase to 180 million by the year 2010 (WHO Study Group 1997).

In a prospective study of 114 281 nurses (Colditz *et al.* 1995) aged 30–55 years who did not have diabetes at the outset, after adjustment for age BMI was the dominant predictor of risk.

Fig 5.3 Impact of obesity on morbidity.

Cardiovascular system	Hypertension
	Coronary heart disease
	Cerebrovascular disease
	Deep vein thrombosis
	Varicose veins
Gastrointestinal system	Hiatus hernia
	Cholelithiasis
	Fatty infiltration of the liver
	Haemorrhoids
	Hernia
Colorectal cancer	Metabolic hyperlipidaemia
	Hyperinsulinism/insulin resistance/type 2 diabetes
Respiratory	Breathlessness
	Sleep apnoea
Pregnancy	Obstetric complications
Musculoskeletal	Osteoarthritis
Breast	Breast cancer
Uterus	Endometrial cancer
	Cervical cancer
Skin	Fungal infections
	Intertrigo
	Cellulitis
	Lymphoedema
Urological	Stress incontinence

In women the risk:

- Rises above a BMI of 22 kg/m^2;
- Increases fivefold at a BMI of 25 kg/m^2;
- Increases 28-fold at a BMI of 30 kg/m^2;
- Increases 93-fold above a BMI of 35 kg/m^2.

A weight gain of 8–10.9 kg gives a 2.7-fold increase in the risk of developing type 2 diabetes compared with those whose weight remains stable.

In a study of 51 529 men aged 40–75 years (Chan *et al.* 1994), there was found to be an increased risk of developing type 2 diabetes above a BMI of 24 kg/m^2. Adjusted for age, the risks were increased:

- twofold at BMI 25–26.9 kg/m^2;
- 6.7-fold at BMI 29–30.9 kg/m^2;
- 42-fold at BMI 35 kg/m^2 or above.

Fat distribution is important and waist circumference was found to be independently associated with the risk of developing type 2 diabetes.

A waist circumference above 100 cm (40 inches) increased the risk 3.5-fold, even after controlling for BMI.

Population studies have dramatically shown the links between obesity and diabetes. Pima Indians of Arizona, Micronesian Nauran islanders and Chinese emigrants to Mauritius are all normally lean individuals and diabetes was a rarity in their natural habitat when they survived at subsistence level. However, with the adoption of sedentary overindulgence of the western lifestyle, obesity has become epidemic (WHO Study Group 1997).

- 80% of adult Pima Indians are obese.
- 40% of adults have type 2 diabetes which rises to 70% in those over 60 years of age (Zimmet 1982).

Distribution of body fat

This is extremely important; over 40 years ago Vague (Vague 1956) pointed out the strong association between android obesity and the development of type 2 diabetes. Nowadays android obesity is recognized as an integral feature of Syndrome X (Metabolic syndrome, Reaven's syndrome) along with hypertension, insulin reistance, hyperinsulinaemia, dyslipidaemia, glucose intolerance, a precoagulant tendency, and accelerated atheroma development with the associated risk of premature death.

Genetic influences

There are strong genetic influences on the development of type 2 diabetes that probably account for up to 80% of the susceptibility to developing the condition (McCarthy *et al.* 1994). In fact, it is likely that common factors, both genetic and environmental, predispose to the development of obesity and diabetes.

Support for this comes from the studies on Pima Indians (referred to above) who in their natural habitat are lean and amongst whom diabetes is virtually unknown.

In fact, in their natural habitat Pima Indians survive at barely subsistence levels and 'thrifty' genes selected during previous struggles to survive under harsh conditions could favour the storage of energy as fat to aid survival through periods of famine. These could act by impairing the action of insulin in skeletal muscle, thus contributing to a degree of insulin resistance. However, when such genetically programmed subjects are exposed to the sedentary overindulgence of the western lifestyle the result is an epidemic of obesity and type 2 diabetes.

Further support for this mechanism comes from the fact that type 2 diabetes is more common in people who are malnourished *in utero* but become obese later in life (Hales *et al.* 1992) (see Fig. 5.4).

Insulin resistance

Under basal conditions, insulin is released in small, regular pulses every 9–12 min (Matthews 1991). Insulin is crucial to many metabolic processes but in the context of obesity and the development of type 2 diabetes, its actions in carbohydrate and fat metabolism are particularly important.

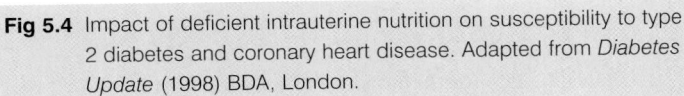

Fig 5.4 Impact of deficient intrauterine nutrition on susceptibility to type 2 diabetes and coronary heart disease. Adapted from *Diabetes Update* (1998) BDA, London.

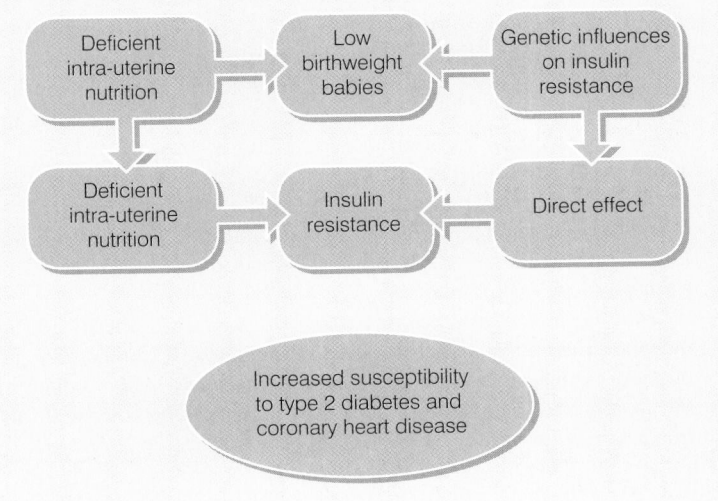

Carbohydrate metabolism

Insulin lowers blood glucose levels by:

- Suppressing the production and secretion of glucose by the liver (gluconeogenesis); in this it is opposed by catecholamines glucagon, growth hormone and cortisol.
- Stimulating the uptake of glucose by skeletal muscle (the most important) and adipose tissue.

Fat metabolism

Insulin inhibits the breakdown of triglyceride (lipolysis) stored in adipose tissue. Lipolysis releases-non-esterified fatty acids (NEFAs) and glycerol (glycerol is a substrate for gluconeogenesis).

Lipolysis is normally very sensitive to inhibition by insulin and is suppressed by relatively low levels of circulating insulin. Lipolysis is strongly stimulated by catecholamines released into the circulation from sympathetic nerve terminals in adipose tissue.

There is some evidence that android adipose tissue is less sensitive to the lipolytic action of insulin and more sensitive to the stimulant action of catecholamines.

As obesity increases, so do the demands on the pancreatic beta cell to produce more insulin, to maintain glucose homeostasis.

Increasing obesity also means an increasing mass of adipose tissue that is increasingly insensitive to the antilypolytic action of insulin. An increasing mass of adipose tissue means more sympathetic nerve terminals to release catecholamines. The result is that lipolysis gains the upper hand and there is the release in increasing amounts of NEFAs, glycerol and TNF from the breakdown of adipocytes.

In the early stages of raised glucose and NEFA levels they have a stimulant action on insulin release, and a resulting hyperinsulinaemia is able to maintain glucose homeostasis; but later, chronically high levels of NEFA interfere with the inhibitory action of insulin on hepatic gluconeogenesis and with the uptake of glucose by skeletal muscle (Pervis *et al.* 1986). Tumour necrosis factor is present in adipose tissue and released by lipolysis and skeletal muscle; it could possibly induce insulin resistance by causing damage to the insulin receptor.

In addition, when high levels of glucose and NEFA are prolonged they impair rather than stimulate beta cell function and lead to the development of frank type 2 diabetes.

There is thus a progressive pattern of increasing obesity leading to increased insulin resistance. As long as the beta cell can increase its production of insulin, a state of glucose homeostasis will be maintained, but at the price of a state of sustained hyperinsulinaemia with all that this brings in its wake.

In addition to impaired glucose tolerance the levels of NEFAs are raised, suggesting insulin insensitivity of the adipose tissue and a degree of failure of insulin to inhibit lipolysis.

Insulin release

There are also deficiencies in insulin release: the first phase of release following food ingestion and stimulation is delayed.

In addition obesity, especially of the android type is associated with increased insulin resistance in the adipocyte and skeletal muscle.

Insulin extraction

Compared with their non-obese counterparts people with android obesity show a decrease in the hepatic extraction of insulin, with the consequence that post-hepatic levels are increased. This could explain the state of hyperinsulinaemia seen in such people (see Fig. 5.5).

Neuroendocrine factors

Recent work from Sweden (Bjorntop *et al.* 1999) suggests a role for the hypothalamo–pituitary–adrenal axis (HPAA), and reports that subjects who lack the normal diurnal variation in cortisol levels have a high prevalence of all the features of the metabolic syndrome.

Although as yet there is no compelling proof (O'Rahilly 1999) of this theoretical model, it should be remembered that:

- acute psychological stress can activate the HPAA;
- life is more stressful for the poor;
- there is compelling evidence that there is a strong association between lower socio-economic class, syndrome X and cardiovascular disease (Brunner *et al.* 1998).

Figure 5.6 summarizes the stages in the development of type 2 diabetes.

In summary, the following factors are important in the development of type 2 diabetes (Fig. 5.7).

Fig 5.5 Relationship of obesity to insulin resistance.

	Gluto Femoral Obesity	Android Obesity
Insulin sensitivity compared to non obese	Down 23%	Down 55%
Insulin secretion compared to non obese	Up 350%	Up 315%

The importance of insulin resistance

The ability of insulin to stimulate the uptake of glucose varies widely between different individuals. In an effort to maintain glucose homeostasis, the pancreatic beta cell will endeavour to produce the amount of insulin necessary to achieve this. The more an individual is insulin resistant, the greater must be the compensatory hyperinsulinaemia.

The defect in insulin action in about 25% of these individuals differs little from those with frank type 2 diabetes. Such individuals are hyperinsulinaemic when compared with an insulin-sensitive control group

Fig 5.6 Stages in the development of type 2 diabetes.

Genetic and environmental factors
Development of obesity
Development of insulin resistance
Compensatory hyperinsulinaemia
Lipotoxicity and glucotoxity
Beta cell failure
Impaired glucose tolerance
Further beta cell failure
Overt type 2 diabetes

Fig 5.7 Factors important in the development of type 2 diabetes.

ORGAN	DEFECT(S)	MEDIATED BY
Liver	Failure of insulin to inhibit gluconeogenesis and glycogenolysis	NEFA, possibly tumour necrosis factor (TNFα)
Skeletal muscle	Impaired insulin-induced uptake of glucose	NEFA, tumour necrosis factor α
Adipocyte (android)	Lipolysis less inhibited by insulin leads to liberation of NEFA and tissue necrosis factor	Resistin
Increasing android adipose tissue	More sympathetic nerve terminals to release catecholamines to stimulate lipolysis	Catecholamines
Pancreatic beta cells	Loss of basal pulsatile release of insulin	? NEFA and tumour necrosis factor, glucotoxity,lipotoxity
Hypothalamo–pituitary–adrenal axis	Lack of diurnal variation in cortisol levels to increased lipolysis	

and it is this hyperinsulinaemia which enables them to maintain glucose homeostasis. 'However, the ability to maintain the degree of compensatory hyperinsulinaemia does not represent an unqualified homeostatic victory' (Reaven 1995). It is bought at a price and that price is the development of syndrome X and an increased risk of developing coronary heart disease.

'*Once chronic food intoxication is recognized by the public as a major cause of type 2 diabetes, preventing and slowing its progress would be considerably helped. To this end the food industry could be strongly regulated to produce a tasty diet, low in saturated fat and of reduced calorie content. For the food industry this could be advisable since it is possible that in the future it could be paying damages similar to the tobacco companies.*' (Waldhausal 2001).

OBESITY AND CARDIOVASCULAR DISEASE

Epidemiological studies show a connection between obesity and cardiovascular disease (CVD). The Nurses' Health Study (Willett *et al.* 1995) showed that the risk of coronary heart disease increased twofold at BMI 25–28.9 and 3.6 times at BMI ≥29. In males the figures are even more convincing, in that a 10% increase in weight gives a 38% increase in the risk of developing coronary heart disease, and a 20% increase in weight gives a staggering 26% increase in risk (RCP 1983).

The Framingham study (Hubert *et al.* 1983), after 26 years of follow-up, confirmed an independent relationship between mild, moderate and severe overweight and increased risk of CVD. Weight gain after the age of 25 appears to have the greater impact on increasing the risk of CVD. Left ventricular hypertrophy—considered to be an ominous risk factor for coronary heart disease, stroke, and cardiac failure—seems to increase with greater BMI at any age; body weight is one of the more powerful determinants of left ventricular size and wall thickness (Lavie *et al.* 1992).

Android obesity is associated with a greater risk of CVD than general obesity; it is also associated with a clustering of risk factors for CVD, including dislipidaemia (high total, and LDL cholesterol with reduced HDL cholesterol), hypertriglyceridaemia, hypertension, insulin resistance, hyperinsulinaemia, glucose intolerance, hypercoagulability, and hypofibrinalyses as described by Reaven (Reaven 1988). It is sometimes referred to as 'the metabolic syndrome, Syndrome X' or 'the chronic cardiovascular risk syndrome'.

Prospective studies (Lapidus *et al.* 1984) have shown a positive association between waist : hip ratio (as a measure of android obesity) and mortality from cardiovascular disease.

Blood pressure

Hypertension is an important risk factor for the development of coronary heart disease and the most important risk factor for stroke. Epidemiological studies have consistently shown that there is a higher prevalence of hypertension in people who are obese (Stamler et al. 1978). In the Framingham study (MacMahon et al. 1987) for each 4.5 kg gain in weight, systolic blood pressure increased by 4.4 mmHg in men and 4.2 mmHg in women.

Obesity is thus a strong independent risk factor for hypertension. In one study the prevalence of hypertension in the obese was estimated to be 50–300% higher than in lean subjects (Stamler et al. 1978). Friedman's longitudinal study (Friedman 1988) showed that weight gain was independently related to increased blood pressure—the extent could be determined by gender ethnicity and age (Hseuh & Buchanan 1994).

Body fat distribution is a more powerful determinant of hypertension, with android obesity being more important than gluteo-femoral.

Hypertension is, of course, an essential component of Reaven's syndrome (referred to previously) and hypertensive individuals appear to be more insulin-resistant than their normotensive counterparts.

Lipid metabolism

Obesity of android distribution is associated with raised levels of triglycerides and LDL cholesterol, and reduced levels of HDL cholesterol, which in turn are part of Reaven's syndrome and increase the risk of developing cardiovascular disease.

Haemostatic factors

Increasing weight gain is associated with rising levels of factors VII and X and increased blood viscosity, which could relate to the risk of thrombosis and fatal myocardial infarction.

OBESITY AND GASTRO-INTESTINAL DISEASE

Gall bladder disease is commonly associated with obesity. In a study of 73 532 obese women in Canada and the USA, Rimm and colleagues reported a 27-fold increase in the prevalence of gall bladder disease (Rimm et al. 1975).

In the Nurses' Health Study (Stampfer et al. 1992) which followed nearly 90 000 women over 8 years, women with a BMI >24 kg/m^2 had a sevenfold excess risk of gallstone disease compared with those with a BMI <24 kg/m^2.

A study of 1224 patients referred for endoscopy (Stene-Larsen 1988) supports the view that obesity is associated with both sliding hiatus hernia and reflux oesophagitis.

There is a well documented association between obesity and liver disorders that range from fatty liver to fatty hepatitis to fatty fibrosis and cirrhosis (Braillon *et al.* 1985). However, most patients show only fatty infiltration. Although a high percentage of morbidly obese patients show histological abnormalities, most remain asymptomatic (Powell *et al.* 1990).

It has been suggested that these changes are part of the insulin resistance syndrome, and that they are independently related to the distribution of fat, and common in those with the android pattern of obesity.

OBESITY AND CANCER

There are differences between pre- and postmenopausal women. It appears that lean women are more at risk of premenopause breast cancer and that there is a higher risk of postmenopausal breast cancer in obese women (Swanson 1989).

One possible explanation is that adipose tissue contains high levels of aromatase, the enzyme that converts androgens into oestrogens: thus the accumulation of adipose tissue in obesity results in a higher oestrogen level. In addition, in obese people there is a reduction in the sex-hormone-binding globulins, which will in turn increase circulating levels of oestrogen.

Endometrial cancer

There are consistent and positive associations between obesity and the incidence of endometrial cancer (Austin *et al.* 1991). The mechanism could well be the same as that in breast cancer.

OBESITY AND RESPIRATORY DISORDERS

Obesity produces a measurable reduction in pulmonary function and has strong associations with sleep apnoea and obesity-related hyperventilation. Sleep disordered breathing has a number of clinical consequences including excess cardiovascular morbidity (Grunstein *et al.* 1993; Grunstein *et al.* 1995).

OBESITY AND PREGNANCY

Obese women have a higher risk of obstetric complication including diabetes hypertension, urinary infection and pre-eclampsia. They also have an increased rate of Caesarean delivery for a number of reasons such as foetal size, soft-tissue narrowing of the birth canal, prolonged labour, intrapartum meconium staining of the liquor, and malpresentations (Garbaciak *et al.* 1985).

After delivery obese women have a higher rate of thrombophlebitis and wound infections.

OBESITY AND ARTHRITIS

There is evidence that obesity is associated with the development of arthritis of the knee and hip.

CONCLUSION

The ramifications of obesity are immense. It is intimately and causally related to the development of some of the major diseases affecting the westernized world, which in turn cause much human suffering and premature loss of life, and place massive economic burdens on society. Obesity is not a simple matter of gluttony or sloth but a major disease of those with a genetic predisposition that is fuelled by today's environment. As such it merits consideration as a disease in its own right.

References

Austin, H., Austin, J., Partridge, E. *et al.* (1991) Endometrial cancer, obesity and body fat distribution. *Cancer Research* **51**, 566–572.

Bjorntop, P., Hom, G. & Rosmond, R. (1999) Hypothalamic arousal, insulin resistance and type 2 diabetes mellitus. *Diabetic Medicine* **16**, 373–381.

Braillon, A., Capion, J.P., Herve, M. *et al.* (1985) Liver in obesity. *Gut* **26**, 133–139.

Brunner, E., Juneja, M. & Marmot, M. (1998) Abdominal obesity and disease linked to social position. *British Medical Journal* **316**, 308–309.

Chan, J.M., Stampfer, M.J., Rimm, E.B. *et al.* (1994) Obesity fat distribution and weight gain as risk factors for clinical diabetes in man. *Diabetes Care* **17**, 961–969.

Colditz, G.A., Willett, W.C., Rotizky, A. *et al.* (1995) Weight gain as a risk factor for clinical diabetes mellitus in women. *Annuals of Internal Medicine* **122**, 481–486.

Friedman, G.D., Selby, J.V., Quesenberry, C.P. *et al.* (1988) Precursors of essential hypertension: body weight, alcohol and salt use, and parental history of hypertension. *Preventative Medicine* **17**, 387–402.

Garbaciak, J.A., Richter, M., Miller, S. *et al.* (1985) Material weight and pregnancy complications. *Annual Journal of Obstetrics and Gynaecology* **152**, 238–245.

Grunstein, R.R., Stenlof, K., Hedner, J.A. & Sjostrom, L. (1995) Impact of sleep apnoea and sleepiness on metabolic and cardiovascular risk factors in the Swedish Obese Subjects (SOS) Study. *International Journal of Obesity* **19**, 410–418.

Grunstein, R.R., Wilcox, I., Yang, T.S., Gould, Y. & Hedner, J.A. (1993) Snoring and sleep apnoea in men: association with central obesity and hypertension. *International Journal of Obesity* **17**, 533–540.

Hales, C.N. & Barker, D.J.P. (1992) Type 2 diabetes mellitus: the thrifty phenotype hypothesis. *Diabetologica* **35**, 595–601.

Herbert, H., Fernlab, M., McNamara, P. *et al.* (1983) Obesity as an independent risk factor for cardiovascular disease. A 26 year follow-up of participants in the Framingham Study. *Circulation* **67**, 968–977.

Hseuh, W. & Buchanan, T. (1994) Obesity and hypertension. *Endocrinology and Metabolism Clinics of North America* **23**, 405–427.

Jung, R.T. (1997) Obesity as a disease. *British Medical Bulletin* **53**, 307–321.

Lapidus, L., Bergtsson, G., Lavvson, B. *et al.* (1984) Distribution of adipose tissue and risk of cardiovascular disease and death. A 12 year follow-up of particpants in the population study of women in Gothenburg, Sweden. *British Medical Journal* **289**, 1257–1261.

Lavie, C., Ventura, H., Messerli, F. (1992) Left ventricular hypertrophy. Its relationship to obesity and hypertension. *Postgraduate Medicine* **91**, 131–143.

Lew, E.A. & Garfinkel, L. (1979) Variations in mortality by weight among 750 000 men and women. *Journal of Chronic Disease* **32**, 563–576.

MacMahon, S., Cutler, J., Brittain, E. *et al.* (1987) Obesity and hypertension: epidemiological and clinical issues. *European Heart Journal* **8** (Suppl. B), 57–70.

Manson, J.E., Willett, W.C., Stampfer, M.J. *et al.* (1995) Body weight and mortality among women. *New England Journal of Medicine* **333**, 677–685.

Matthews, D.R. (1991) Physiological implications of pulsalite hormone secretion. *Annals of the New York Academy of Science* **618**, 28–37.

McCarthy, M.G., Frogue, P. & Hitzman, G.A. (1994) The genetics of non insulin dependent diabetes mellitus: tools and aims. *Diabetologia* **37**, 959–968.

O'Rahilly, S. (1999) The metabolic syndrome: all in the mind? *Diabetic Medicine* **16**, 355–356.

Pervis, A.N., Mueller, R.A., Smith, G.A. *et al.* (1986) Splanchinic insulin metabolism in obesity—influence of body fat distribution. *Journal of Clinical Investigation* **78**, 1648–1657.

Powell, E., Cockstey, G., Hanson, R. *et al.* (1990) The natural history of non alcoholic steatohepatitis: a follow-up study of forty two patients up to 21 years. *Hepatology* **11**, 4–80.

RCS. (1983) Obesity. *Journal Royal College of Physicians* **17**, 3–58.

Reaven, G.M. (1995) Pathophysiology of insulin resistance in human disease. *Physiological Review* **75** (3), 473–486.

Reaven, G.M. (1988) Role of insulin resistance in human disease. *Diabetes* **37**, 1595–1607.

Rimm, A.A., Weiner, L.H., Van Ysortoo, B. *et al.* (1975) Relationship of obesity and disease in 73 532 weight conscious women. *Public Health Report* **90**, 44–51.

Stamler, R., Stamler, J., Riedlinger, W.F. *et al.* (1978) Weight and blood pressure. Findings in hypertension screening of 1 million Americans. *Journal of the Americam Medical Association* **240**, 1607–1610.

Stampfer, M., McClure, K., Colditz, G. *et al.* (1992) Risk of symptomatic gallstones in women with severe obesity. *American Journal of Clinical Nutrition* **55**, 652–658.

Stene-Larsen, G., Weberg, R., Froyshov Larsen, I. *et al.* (1988) Relationship of overweight to hiatus hernia and reflux oesophagitis. *Scandinavian Journal of Gastroenterology* **23**, 427–432.

Swanson, C.A., Coates, R.J., Schoenberg, J.B. *et al.* (1996) Body size and breast cancer risk among women under 45 years of age. *American Journal of Epidemiology* **143**, 698–706.

Vague, J. (1956) The degree of masculine differentiatiom of obesities, a factor determining predisposition to diabetes, atherosclerosis, gout and uric calculous disease. *American Journal of Clinical Nutrition* **4**, 20–34.

Waldhausal, W.K. (2001) Finally we have arrived in the new millenium. *Diabetologia* **44**, 1–2.

WHO Study Group. (1994) *Prevention of Diabetes Mellitus*. WHO Technical Report Series; 844.

WHO Study Group. (1997). WHO Technical Report Series.

Willett, W.C., Manson, J.E., Stampfer, M.J. *et al.* (1995) Weight, weight change and coronary heart disease in women. *Journal of the Americam Medical Association* **27**, 1461–1465.

Zimmet, P. (1982) Type 2 diabetes mellitus–an epidemiological overview. *Diabetologia* **22**, 399–411.

6 Beneficial effects of modest weight loss

INTRODUCTION

As has been shown previously, moderate to severe obesity increases both mortality and morbidity risks particularly those associated with type 2 diabetes, vascular disease and certain cancers. However, even though the beneficial effects of weight reduction are widely known, obese people find if difficult to achieve optimal body weight and even greater difficulty in sustaining it (Kaplan & Atkina 1987).

Perhaps the most important discovery of recent years in the management of obesity has been the impact of a 5–10% weight loss in terms of improving an individual's risk profile (Blackburn & Kandera 1987). This is a goal which, for many, is both achievable and sustainable and can have a major impact in reducing the mortality and morbidity associated with obesity.

MORTALITY

- A weight loss of more than 9 kg in obese women is associated with a 25% reduction in all-cause mortality (Williamson et al. 1995).
- If the obese person already has an obesity-related disease, intentional weight loss can reduce mortality by 20%. This is most marked for cancer (30–40%) and for diabetes (30–40% fall in mortality).

TYPE 2 DIABETES

- A weight loss of 5 kg reduces the risk of developing diabetes by more than 50% (Manson et al. 1995).
- A 9-kg weight loss reduces diabetes-related mortality by 30–40% (Williamson et al. 1995).
- A 5% weight loss reduces HbAIC by 7% and fasting blood glucose by 15% (Dattilo & Kria-Etherton 1992).
- A weight loss of 10–20% in people with type 2 diabetes can normalize metabolic control and significantly improve life expectancy (Jung 1997).

CARDIOVASCULAR DISEASE

Weight loss affects the five (modifiable) principal risk factors of CVD.

- Hypertension.
- Hyperlipidaemia.
- Type 2 diabetes and insulin resistance.
- Haemostatic factors.
- Rheological factors.
    Each will be dealt with in turn.

Hypertension
- A weight loss of 11 kg produced a 20% decrease in both systolic and diastolic pressures (Reisen *et al.* 1978).
- As a general rule, blood pressure is reduced by 1 mm systolic and 2 mm diastolic for each 1% reduction in weight (Jung 1997).
- It is clear that in clinical practice a weight loss of 5–10 kg will produce a valuable reduction in blood pressure (Lean *et al.* 1998).

Hyperlipidaemia
- Each kilogram of weight loss reduces total plasma cholesterol and LDL cholesterol by 1%.
- Each kilogram of weight loss increases HDL cholesterol by 1–2%.
- Each kilogram of weight loss reduces triglycerides by 2–3% (Lean & Hankey 1998).

Type 2 diabetes and hyperinsulinaemia
Significant weight loss improves glucose control in patients with type 2 diabetes and ameliorates the associated dyslipidemia, reducing the risk of cardiovascular disease (Wing *et al.* 1987). As has been shown previously there are individuals in a state of glucose homeostasis by courtesy of being in a state of hyperinsulinaemia with its attendant risks of vascular disease.

Haemostatic factors
- A weight reducing diet in 114 overweight subjects for 3 months showed significant falls in the levels of coagulation factors VII and X. Some of this reduction could be related to the reduction in the dietary fat content of the diet.
- Weight loss in obese subjects improves fibrinolysis (Anderson *et al.* 1988), the probable mechanism is the reduction of plasminogen activator factor.

Rheology
For each 2 kg of weight loss there is a:
- 2.5% decrease in red cell aggregation; and
- 2% reduction in plasma viscosity (Lean & Hankey 1998).
    A 15% weight loss was associated with a:

- 27% decrease in blood viscosity; and
- 20% decrease in red cell aggregation (Ernst & Matrai 1987).

The above changes taken together are probably responsible for the improvements in cardiovascular mortality and morbidity.

OSTEOARTHRITIS

A study in people with morbid obesity (BMI > 35 kg/m^2) showed improvements in pain in the lower back, ankles and feet with a 6–10 kg weight loss (McGoey et al. 1990).

RESPIRATORY DISORDERS

Weight loss in the obese improves:
- general measures of pulmonary function;
- sleep apnoea.

IS LOSING WEIGHT HAZARDOUS TO HEALTH?

The answer is most certainly that any health hazards associated with losing weight are vastly outweighed by the benefits.

Most of the health hazards have been associated with the use of very low calorie diets (VLCD) which are not advocated in this text and should only be used in exceptional circumstances in highly specialized inpatient units.

LOSS OF LEAN BODY MASS

Until quite recently the goal of achieving *ideal* body weight did carry with it the hazard of losing lean muscle as well as adipose tissue. This in turn resulted in greater tiredness on exercise thereby prejudicing the achievement of increased physical activity as a key component of weight loss and weight maintenance programmes. The modern approach of seeking more modest weight loss should not significantly affect lean body mass.

CHOLELITHIASIS

Weight loss is associated with an increased risk of developing gallstone disease. In a comprehensive review of the evidence (Everhart 1993) it was found that:
- After weight loss through dietary intervention the development of gall-stones increased by up to 22%.
- Above a weight loss of 24% the risk of gallstone disease increased three-fold.

- When weight losses exceed 45% it is likely that 60% of patients will develop gallstones (Shiffman *et al.* 1991).

It has to be emphasized that the current targets are a 5–10% weight loss which is far less than the percentages quoted above. Nevertheless clinicians must be honest with patients and acknowledge the increased risk of gallstone development while emphasizing that weight loss significantly reduces operative risk.

MECHANISM

It is likely that the increased mobilization of cholesterol from adipose tissue during weight loss leads to the supersaturation of bile which in turn favours the development of gallstones.

BONE MASS

This is responsive to changes in body mass and some loss of bone mass is associated with weight loss and weight maintenance programmes. Using modern targets of 5–10% weight loss is unlikely to put patients at significant risk of developing osteoporosis.

References

Anderson, P., Nilsen, D.W.T., Backkannin, S.H. *et al.* (1988) Increased fibrimolytic potential in healthy coronary high risk individuala. *Acta Medica Scandinavica* **22**, 499–506.

Blackburn, G.L. & Kandera, B.S. (1987) Medical evaluation and treatment of the obese patient with cardiovascular disease. *American Journal of Cardiology* **60**, 556–589.

Dattilo, A.M. & Kria-Etherton, P.M. (1992) Effects of weight reduction on blood lipids and lipoproteins: a meta analysis. *American Journal of Clinical Nutrition* **56**, 320–328.

Ernst, E. & Matrai, A. (1987) Normalisation of hemorrheological abnormalities during weight reduction in obese patients. *Nutrition* **3**, 337–339.

Everhart, J.E. (1993) Contributions of obesity and weight loss to gallstone disease. *Annals of Internal Medicine* **119**, 1029–1035.

Jung, R. (1997) Obesity as a disease. *British Medical Bulletin* **53**, 307–321.

Kaplan, R.M. & Atkins, C.J. (1987) Selective attrition causes overestimates of treatment effects in studies of weight loss. *Addictive Behaviour* **12**, 297–302.

Lean, M.E.J. & Hankey, C.R. (1998) Benefits and risks of weight loss: obesity and weight cycling. In: Kopelman PG, Stock MJ (eds) *Clinical Obesity*. pp. 564–596. Blackwell Science: Oxford.

McGoey, B.V., Deitel, M., Saplya, R.J.F *et al.* (1990) Effect of weight loss on musculoskeletal pain in the morbidly obese. *Journal of Bone and Joint Surgery* **72**, 322–323.

Manson, J.E., Willett, W.C., Stampfer, M.J. *et al.* (1995) Body weight and mortality among women. *New England Journal of Medicine* **333**, 677–685.

Reisen, E., Abel, R., Modan, M. *et al.* (1978) The effect of weight loss without salt restriction on the reduction in blood pressure in overweight hypertensive patients. *New England Journal of Medicine* **298**, 1–6.

Shiffman, M.L., Lugerhian, H.J., Kollman, J.M. *et al.* (1991) Gallstone formation after rapid weight loss: a prospective study in patients undergoing gastric bypass surgery for treatment of morbid obesity. *American Journal of Gastroenterology* **86**, 1000–1005.

Williamson, D.F., Pamuk, E., Thun, M. *et al.* (1995) Prospective Study of intentional weight loss and mortality in never smoking overweight US white women aged 40–64 years. *American Journal of Epidemiology* **141**, 1128–1124.

Wing, R.R., Koeske, R., Epstein, L.H. *et al.* (1987) Long term effects of modest weight loss in type 2 diabetic patients. *Archives of Internal Medicine* **147**, 1749–1753.

Management in clinical practice: a patient orientated approach

'Effective weight management does not simply mean organizing a slimming process… it is a completely different concept geared to ensuring that the long-term health of the patient is the key concern' (James 1998).

Obese people are often discriminated against socially and tend to have low self-esteem. Researchers have documented negative attitudes and bias among family doctors, nurses and medical students. Such negative attitudes by health professionals will only served to reinforce patients' negative stereotypes about obesity and are likely to deter them from seeking help.

Fig 7.1 Setting the tone: how to communicate with patients.

• Empathic	vs	unconcerned
• Unbiased	vs	judgmental
• Supportive	vs	dismissive
• Accepting	vs	fault-finding
• Optimistic	vs	sceptical

Although obesity does result from an imbalance between energy intake and expenditure it is not a simple matter of gluttony or sloth! (Prentice & Jebb 1995) and is not as much self-inflicted or as much under the sphere of control as many have previously thought.

Given that obesity can markedly reduce both lifespan and the quality of life through its association with coronary heart disease, diabetes, certain cancers, respiratory problems and musculoskeletal disorders, surely it is worth regarding it as a condition worthy of medical attention and treating people who are obese with the same compassion that we would wish to show to people with cancer. In 1927 Sir Francis Peabody said: 'The significance of the intimate personal relationship between physician and patient cannot be too strongly emphasized, for in an extraordinarily large number of cases both diagnosis and treatment depend directly upon it and the failure of the young physician to establish this relationship accounts for much of his ineffectiveness in the care of patients.' This has more latterly been seen in terms of patient-centred consultations which is really a shift from thinking about patient care in terms of disease and pathology to thinking in terms of people and their problems (Henbest & Stewart 1990).

Obesity is undoubtedly one of the most challenging conditions to be managed in primary care today but success is more likely if obese patients are treated with understanding and respect.

To begin with it should be established whether the patient is prepared to be committed to a weight loss and weight maintenance programme, which to gain maximum benefit, is likely to have to be pursued for the rest of that person's life. Without a degree of such commitment, success is unlikely and the result likely to be the waste of a considerable amount of time by both doctor and patient. Here it is worth taking time to emphasize that what is being sought is not necessarily ideal body weight (a daunting prospect) but the loss of 5–10% or 10 kg which is realistically achievable by most people.

The benefits of such a weight loss should be emphasized in terms of likely increased longevity and better quality of life from the reduced risk of developing coronary heart disease, diabetes, certain cancers, respiratory problems and musculoskeletal disorders, and not least, improved self-image and esteem.

- Identify the high-risk, obese patient—define severity of obesity, fat distribution and comorbidities.
- Assess targets of opportunity for intervention and readiness for change.
- Initiate treatment and provide management for obesity and comorbidities.
- Use referral sources (team) as indicated. (Kushner 1998).

If commitment is forthcoming it is worth taking a brief dietary and exercise history and making an evaluation of mental status. It is also worth reviewing previous attempts at weight loss, the degree of success achieved, and what the patient weighed two to three years after each attempt.

Doctors should be aware that some patients will have in the past lost and gained hundreds of pounds following weight loss programmes and will undoubtedly be blaming themselves for their lack of success. Before resorting to dietary manipulation, it is worth establishing a patient's eating habits by the keeping of a food diary for four to six weeks. Many obese people do not believe that they eat abnormally or excessively and there is no substitute for precise data collection. The doctor should be honest about the difficulties of weight loss and weight maintenance and encourage the patient to set realistic and achievable goals. It should be acknowledged that achieving significant weight loss and control exacts a cost which can be quite high in terms of time, attention and sacrifice but that the awards are considerable.

WHO SHOULD BE TARGETTED?

The prevalence is so great that primary care workers will have to be selective and target their activities on priority groups:
- Those who are motivated—without motivation the investment of time by the patient and by the clinician is likely to be wasted.
- Those with obesity related conditions.
- Those with a BMI ≥30 kg/m^2 with comorbid risk factors.
- Those with a BMI ≥30 kg/m^2 with a close family history of type 2 diabetes and/or premature coronary heart disease in a first degree relative.
- Women who remain overweight after pregnancy.

Groups not to target are as follows:
- Those not motivated as this will be a waste of valuable time.
- Pregnant women.
- Breast feeding mothers.
- Elderly people who are obese but otherwise healthy.

ORGANIZATION OF SERVICES

It has previously been argued that obesity is a chronic disease in its own right, worthy of the same attention currently given to other chronic conditions, e.g. asthma and diabetes. People with chronic diseases are increasingly offered not only diagnosis and therapy, but also continued support and structured follow-up. Most clinicians would find it indefensible to diagnose hypertension and offer therapy without continued support and surveillance.

If obesity is accepted as a disease in its own right as was argued in Chapter 5, then surely it merits a similar approach to its management as is afforded to other chronic conditions. While the ideal would be for diagnosis and management to lie with the primary healthcare teams, in some areas the sheer size of the problem coupled with the workloads shouldered by primary care teams would make this an impossible goal to achieve. In these circumstances, Primary Care Organizations could consider the development of a centre to serve the needs of the Group, staffed by appropriately trained clinicians who would take referrals from primary healthcare teams. Work on obesity could be combined with work on smoking cessation as smoking is also worthy of considering as a disease in its own right. Facilities could well be housed in the planned Health Living Centres and become a valued community resource.

Obese patients with other obesity related conditions clearly merit quite intensive treatment and support. There will remain a further group who appear, apart from their obesity, to be otherwise healthy. Whether they remain so largely depends on whether or not they are insulin resistant. Unfortunately, the means do not exist at present to easily measure insulin resistance so that it is necessary to identify other markers which, if present, strongly suggest its presence. These are android obesity, mildly raised triglycerides, slightly lowered HDL, raised uric acid and borderline hypertension which, clustered together, are markers of syndrome X and indicate that those with them are at significantly greater risk of developing accelerated atheroma, coronary heart disease and type 2 diabetes.

People in this category also merit intensive treatment and support. Those obese people without such markers are likely to be the ones who will live a normal life-span without intensive interventions.

CHANGING PATIENTS' EXPECTATIONS AND GOALS

Most obese people have unrealistic expectations about the amount of weight they can lose and their ability to maintain their new weight.

For too long a return to the so called ideal body weight has been considered by the medical profession to be both a possible and mandatory target for obese people. This misconception has been transmitted to the public, and has been reinforced by the media's promotion of slenderness as the ideal body image.

'There is now considerable pressure on the overweight individual to return to his/her ideal, often within the lower end of the normal (18.5–25 kg/m^2) BMI range' (IOTF 1998).

Returning to an ideal body weight is not an appropriate goal and is considered to be counter productive for the following reasons as set out by the International Obesity Task Force (IOTF 1998):

1   Substantial benefit, such as a 25% decline in mortality, can accrue from modest weight losses of 5–10 kg in one year.
2   Physiological responses limit weight loss, so it is unusual to return to normal weight.
3   Clinical trials show that many patients are unable to continue losing weight for longer than 12–16 weeks (4–8 kg loss) and that weight loss does not continue past 6 months.
4   Repeated failures to achieve and sustain substantial weight loss may amplify a patient's depression and lack of self esteem and may result in further weight gain.
5   Long-term health depends on limiting weight gain over a period of years.

It is important to recognize the differences between the expectations of patients and clinicians in weight management. A realistic goal is the loss of 5–10% (10 kg) of body weight and then the maintenance of the resultant body weight over a period of many years (Figs 7.2 & 7.3).

Fig 7.2 Differences between the expectations of patient and physician in weight management.

	Patient	Physician
Rate of weight loss	quick	progressive
Level of weight loss (% of initial weight)	20%	5–10%
Diet duration	some weeks	rest of life
Goals	weight loss	weight maintenance
	cosmetic purposes	to decrease obesity comorbidities
	physical fitness	metabolic fitness

Fig 7.3 Unrealistic goals: average fashion model vs average woman.

	Average fashion model	Average woman
Height	5'9"	5'4"
Weight	110 lb	142 lb
BMI	16.3 kg/m^2	24.4 kg/m^2

DIETARY MANAGEMENT

Principles

1 National food surveys indicate that obesity levels have increased and this has been mirrored by an increase in the proportion of fat intake and a decrease in carbohydrate intake. Three facts are of major importance:

- One gram of fat yields 9 kilocalories, 1 gram of carbohydrate yields 4 kilocalories.
- Energy intake from fat is more easily converted into body fat than that from carbohydrate.
- High-fat foods are often extremely palatable but less filling than those high in carbohydrate.

Thus a diet for weight loss and weight maintenance should be high in carbohydrate and low in fat. In recent years many studies have pointed out that, even without any change in total calorie intake, reducing the percentage of fat in the diet leads to a progressive weight reduction in obese people despite maintaining, or even increasing, the carbohydrate content of the diet. An increase in the carbohydrate content of the diet has been shown to decrease the fat content (Barkhill *et al.* 1996) and WHO now advocate increasing carbohydrate intake to at least 55% of total energy expenditure for the whole population above two years of age.

A major aim is to reduce body fat rather than lean tissue. Garrow (1992) suggests that if weight loss exceeds 1 kg/week this could involve the loss of lean tissue. If this happens it has implications for metabolic rate as the level at which resting metabolic rate is set is determined by the quantity of lean tissue present. If the BMI falls then the energy requirements also fall making it more difficult to sustain weight loss or maintain weight at the desired level.

Drastic reduction in the calorie content has two major disadvantages:

- The loss of lean tissue referred to above.
- Is not an aid to long-term compliance which is essential to a successful weight loss and weight management programme.

While traditionally dietitians have tended to recommend diets of 1000 kcals for women and 1200 kcals for men, over the past few years they have adopted a more flexible approach with small energy reductions with a resulting improvement in compliance and sustained weight loss (Frost 1991).

2 If dietary management is to make an effective and long-term contribution to weight loss and weight maintenance then diets must be palatable, give reasonable feelings of satiety and be capable of being followed long-term. Here it is encouraging to note that diets which are low in fat, but high in carbohydrate compared with traditional low energy diets achieved equal weight loss, but were rated to be more palatable, achieve greater satiety and improve the quality of life (Shah et al. 1994). The conclusion must be that such diets are more likely to be acceptable and capable of making a long-term contribution to weight loss and weight management programmes.

3 Diets must be hypocaloric, but need to make an individual patient's struggle with appetite-drive achievable. Nowadays it is generally agreed that a hypocaloric diet must create a 50–100 kcal/day deficit in relation to total daily energy requirements estimated on the basis of BMR and physical activity. Very low calorie diets tend to induce intensive compensatory drives to eat and are often associated with later weight gain. Prescribing an individualized hypocaloric diet based on an estimate of energy expenditure is more likely to achieve success than prescribing a standard low calorie diet. This has been demonstrated in clinical practice (Lean & James 1986) which showed that obese people with type 2 diabetes on a diet of 1600 kilocalories per day lost significantly more weight than those on a diet of 1200 kilocalories per day (Fig. 7.4).

4 There are no miracle diets!

5 Each obese person should be evaluated carefully in order to individualize the diet to his or her particular necessities and gastronomic preferences.

Fig 7.4 Characteristics of a correct hypocaloric diet (Formiguera 1999).

* Contain at least the minimal daily requirements of macro- and micronutrients
* Be palatable, maintaining the 'hedonistic' value of food
* Take into account the type of work and the time schedule
* Consider age, pregnant status, etc.
* Avoid absolute prohibitions

Who should give dietary advice?

The identification of people with a body mass of $30 \, kg/m^2$ and with a family history of type 2 diabetes and/or prevalence of premature coronary heart disease in a first degree relative, or with a BMI of $27 \, kg/m^2$ with obesity-related conditions, is likely to be by members of primary healthcare teams. Such members should be able to give advice based on the general principles of dietary management outlined above and illustrated in Fig. 7.5. Thereafter, referrals should be made to a dietician for individualized dietary advice. See also 'Organization of services, p.49'.

Success is more likely if:

* The whole family is involved (Cousins *et al.* 1992).
* Change is introduced gradually.
* The patient receives individualized advice.
* Changes are negotiated rather than imposed.
* Realistic targets are set as staging posts along the path of weight reduction.

Counselling on diet

If counselling is to be effective it must be:

* Accurate—advice must be based on hard facts not guess work.
* Practical—so that it can enable patients to relate to their own eating habits.
* Realistic—within the recipient's lifestyle.
* Meaningful—simple to understand and relevant to the problem being discussed.
* Affordable—many nutritional problems are more prevalent in the lower socio-economic groups.
* Accessible—a phone helpline may be more effective than waiting several days for a clinic appointment and the provision of essential advice.

Very low calorie diets

Very low calorie diets (VLCDO) really have no place other than in specialized centres for the management of obese people who urgently need to lose weight.

Fig 7.5 A guide to healthier eating.

Increasing starches

Wholemeal Bread

Porridge or high fibre wholegrain cereals

Potatoes, pasta or rice

Include pulses and vegetables in meat dishes

Wholemeal flour in baking

Decreasing fat

Avoid frying

Choose lean cuts

Trim off visible fat

Don't add meat fat to gravies

Avoid pies and sausages

Cook in vegetable oil which is changed frequently

Low fat polyunsaturated margarines

Decreasing sugars

Decrease use in cooking and at table

Artificial sweeteners

Fresh or dried fruit can add sweetness to taste

Low calorie or sugar free drinks

Avoid confectionery

Increasing fruit/vegetables

Increase use of wider range in salads

Two vegetables at each meal

Fruit as a desert instead of puddings

Bowls of fruit on display for easy access

Include vegetables in meat dishes, e.g. stews and curries

Decreasing salt

Fresh food in preference to tinned or packaged

Use more herbs and spices to add flavour

Minimum use in cooking and at table

Reduce meat and vegetable extracts

They are unsuitable for the following categories of people (DHSS 1987). Those with:

- Heart disease.
- Kidney disease.
- Hypertension.
- Cancer.
- Diabetes treated with insulin.
- Sulphonylurea drugs.
- Porphyria or gout and the following:
  (i)   pregnant and breast feeding women;
  (ii)   children;
  (iii) adolescents;
  (iv)   elderly population.

Assessing diet

Before giving dietary advice, it is essential to know an individual's current eating habits and favourite foods. Here a daily food diary can be useful and an example is given in Fig. 7.6.

The person is asked to write down all they eat and drink over a period of three or four days which includes at least one weekend day.

This helps to identify the types of food eaten and eating patterns as well as providing a reasonable idea of nutritional intake and adequacy of the diet. It also increases self-awareness.

A disadvantage is that when it is known that food intake is to be

Fig 7.6 Example of a food diary.

	Mon	Tue	Wed	Thu	Fri	Sat	Sun
Breakfast	Small bowl of branflakes with semi-skimmed milk, no sugar, coffee with semi-skimmed milk						
During the morning	Apple, coffee with semi-skimmed milk						
Lunch	Cheese and pickle sandwich (granary bread), packet of plain crisps						
During the afternoon	Tea with semi-skimmed milk						
Evening meal	Grilled fish in breadcrumbs, 2 small boiled potatoes, peas, 2 scoops ice cream. Tea with semi-skimmed milk						
Evening snacks	Small packet of peanuts, coffee with semi-skimmed milk						
Alcohol	Pint of lager						

recorded, it can modify eating habits and because people may feel guilty about eating say a packet of potato crisps, this is not recorded. Therefore, it is important that the person is reassured that the purpose of their keeping a record of food intake is not for the professional to pass judgement but for the giving of realistic and appropriate advice.

An alternative method of obtaining information about a person's eating habits, is by the use of a food-frequency questionnaire which can if necessary be completed in advance of the consultation.

Such a questionnaire gathers information about typical eating habits over a period of time and can be assessed by computer software. Certain packages can both assess food intake and provide advice on dietary modification.

Making dietary changes

This can be done by the 'four food group' approach on healthy eating. The food groups are illustrated in Fig. 7.7 and all will provide a variety of essential nutrients.

Foods which are not included, e.g. cakes, biscuits, pies and fizzy drinks, are poor sources of essential nutrients and some are relatively high in saturated fat. They are best excluded from the diet or only eaten occasionally as a 'treat'. It is important that the bulk of the person's diet is selected from the four main food groups.

In moderation foods such as cooking oils and low-fat spreads make the diet more palatable because they provide a source of essential fatty acids.

Within the choices from the four groups it is important that the bulk of the diet comes from cereals and fruit and vegetable groups, and that at least some of the servings are high in non-starch fibre. In the meat and dairy products groups, low-fat choices such as lean meat and low-fat milk and spreads are preferred.

Within each of the four groups it is possible to achieve a variety of choices to avoid a diet that is boring and repetitive, which in turn discourages compliance. Figure 7.8 gives suggestions for modifying the intakes of starch, fibre (NSP), fat, sugar and milk.

A number of studies have shown that calorie-for-calorie fat is more fattening than carbohyrdate and that a high-fat diet predisposes to overweight and obesity, independently of calorie intake, partly by influencing appetite control (Bolton-Smith & Woodward 1993).

The metabolism of protein makes only a small contribution to energy intake so that weight is primarily influenced by the metabolism of carbohyrdate and fat (Jequier 1994).

If energy intake and expenditure match, then weight can be maintained at a stable level even though intakes of carbohyrdate and fat vary. However, if intake exceeds expenditure, a high-fat diet is more likely to lead to weight gain.

Fig 7.7 Food groups.

Bread, cereals and potatoes

Bread: all types including wholemeal, granary, mixed grain, pitta bread, ciabatta bread, French bread, bagel, chapatti, naan

Breakfast cereals

Rice, pasta, noodles

Potato, sweet potato, yam, cassava, (bammie-cassava bread), dasheen oats, maize, cornmeal, polenta, rye, semolina, tapioca, millet, burghul wheat, buckwheat (kasha), barley

Have at least four servings from this group each day and include some high fibre choices.

Examples of a serving:
- A bowl of cereal
- A portion of oats or porridge
- Bread as a sandwich
- Bread with a meal

Milk, cheese and yoghurt

Milk: skimmed, semi-skimmed, whole

Cheese: all types, especially lower fat varieties of hard and soft cheeses

Yoghurt: plain and fruit, and low fat varieties; fromage frais

Have three different servings each day from this group and include low fat choices.

Examples of a serving:
- A glass of milk, e.g. semi-skimmed
- Milk on cereal
- Milk with tea/coffee throughout the day
- A carton of yogurt or fromage frais
- A portion of cheese

Fruit and vegetables

All vegetables, including salad and frozen vegetables (excluding potatoes)

All fresh and frozen fruit (choose fruit in natural juice or water); unsweetened fruit juice

Have at least four different servings each day from this group.

Examples of a serving:
- A piece of fruit, e.g. apple, orange
- A portion of vegetables, e.g. peas, cabbage, mixed vegetables
- A green or mixed salad
- A glass of unsweetened fruit juice
- A bowl of fruit salad

Meat, fish, poultry, eggs, pulses, nuts

Poultry: chicken, turkey, duck

Meat: beef, lamb, pork (including lean bacon), low fat sausages/beefburgers, liver, kidney, rabbit

Fish: white fish, e.g. cod, plaice

Oily fish: e.g. mackerel, tuna, salmon, shellfish

Eggs

Nuts and nut butters, e.g. peanut butter

Pulses: e.g. lentils, dahl, kidney beans, chick peas, baked beans, etc, and products made from these, e.g. tofu, hummus, textured vegetable protein (TVP)

Seeds: sunflower, sesame, pumpkin

Have two servings each day from this group and include low fat choices.

Examples of a serving:
- A portion of lean meat
- A portion of poultry (without skin) or fish
- A portion of shellfish
- An egg or egg dish
- A portion of beans, tofu, nuts or seeds
- A portion of a nut-based dish

Fig 7.8 Suggestions for modifying intakes of starch, fibre (NSP), fat, sugar and milk.

Ways to eat more starch:

- Eat plenty of cereal products such as bread of all kinds, breakfast cereals, rice, pasta, noodles, semolina, tapioca.
- Try grains such as bulgar (cracked) wheat, barley, millet, oats, rye, cornmeal, buckwheat.
- Eat more root vegetables and starchy fruits such as potatoes, yams, cassava, plantain, green bananas.

Ways to eat more NSP:

- Eat plenty of bread, especially wholemeal.
- Try wholemeal pasta and brown rice.
- Where possible choose wholegrain breakfast cereals.
- Eat more vegetables—fresh, frozen or tinned.
- Use more beans and lentils (pulses).
- Eat more potatoes and leave the skin on. Turnips, swedes, cassava, yam and plantain are also good sources of fibre.
- Try using flours such as buckwheat flour or cornmeal in cooking. Mixed 50% : 50% with ordinary flour, buckwheat flour makes excellent pancakes.
- Whole grains, e.g. pearl barley or oats, and pulses can be added to stews and casseroles. Oats can be added to crumble toppings and stuffings.

Reducing fat intake can be relatively easy if a few guidelines are followed:

- Use as little oil or fat as possible when food is prepared or cooked.
- Use spreads sparingly. Butter and margarine contain the same amount of fat and calories – only low fat spreads contain less.
- Cut down on fried foods, such as crisps, and foods that contain a lot of fat but are generally less nourishing, such as greasy snack foods.
- Trim off all the visible fat from meat. Choose lean cuts and grill rather than fry.
- Use low fat alternatives to traditional meat products such as sausages or beefburgers.
- Use semi-skimmed milk, low fat cheese, low fat yogurt or fromage frais.
- Choose low fat snacks, e.g. fruit, currant buns, cereal with low fat milk, low fat yogurts, dried fruit, plain popcorn.
- Eat fewer cakes, pastries, confectionery, and biscuits, as these can contribute considerable amounts of fat.

Fig 7.8 *continued.*

Ways to cut down on sugar:
- Cut down on confectionery, biscuits and cakes.
- Choose low calorie or 'diet' varieties of soft drinks.
- Don't add sugar to tea, coffee and breakfast cereals – most people find they can do without it.
- Cut down on the amount of sugar used in recipes and choose unsweetened breakfast cereals.
- Use unsweetened fruit juices and buy tinned fruit in natural juice rather than in syrup.
- When buying processed foods, look for those that say 'no added sugar'.
- Use honey and jam sparingly.

Ways of cutting down on salt:
- Use fewer salty, processed foods and more fresh or unprocessed foods, which will be naturally lower in salt, e.g. home-made soup rather than packet or tinned soup. When processed foods are purchased, look on the ingredients labels for those with 'no added salt'.
- When selecting snack foods, choose snacks that are not salty, for example: fruit, vegetable sticks, a sandwich or current bun, a yogurt, or raisins and unsalted nuts.
- Use less salt in cooking by flavouring dishes with alternatives such as herbs, spices, lemon juice, or mustard.
- Gradually get used to the taste of food without salt. Taste food before salt is added at the table.

This is because if intake of carbohydrate exceeds requirements, the excess is oxidized readily and in preference to fat. If on the other hand, intake of fat exceeds requirements, people prone to obesity do not have the ability to increase fat oxidation to burn off the excess which then enters their fat stores which are potentially limitless (Jequier 1994).

Physical activity

Promoting physical activity is an essential part of any weight-management programme. Brisk walking and cycling can increase energy expenditure by an extra 60–200 kcal/h in obese and over-weight patients who are normally sedentary. The benefits of physical activity can be seen in Fig. 7.9.

Three hours of daily activity involving standing and not sitting increases the 24-h energy output from 40% to more than 74% above the basal metabolic rate (James & Schofield 1990).

Fig 7.9 Benefits of physical activity.

1 Physical activity is one of the best predictors of success in weight maintenance after a period of weight loss.
2 Improves physical fitness
3 Stimulates fat oxidation
4 Improves the sensitivity to insulin
5 Improves the lipid profile
6 Reduces blood pressure
7 Reduces the risk of sudden death
8 Increases energy expenditure
9 Protects lean body mass
10 Improves psychological factors
11 May suppress appetite

Adapted from Sarvis (1998).

Physical activity is one of the most powerful influences to change metabolism towards successful long-term weight control which is the patient's greatest challenge. All physical activity counts, there is no threshold of activity necessary for benefit.

- All physical activity counts.
- Walk instead of taking the car or bus; 30 min brisk walking will burn 144 calories.
- Park the car further away from the destination to give an opportunity for walking—the Almighty did not design the left foot for the clutch and the right foot for the accelerator!
- Take the stairs instead of the escalator or lift.
- Walk around the shopping mall before buying.
- Switch off the television and go for a walk.
- Walk with a friend (man's best friend is his dog).
- Exercise the family way—swimming, hiking, dancing.
- Improve the garden—even moderately active gardening will expend 50 kcal more than watching television.

Increasing physical activity is not about buying jogging suits and trainers; it is about walking briskly for 20–30 min every day!

References

Barkill, S., Kivk, T.R., Cursiter, M. *et al*. (1996) The potential of starch rich foods in achieving national targets for dietary fat reduction. *Proceedings of the Nutrition Society* **54**, 20.

Bolton-Smith, C. & Woodward, M. (1993) The prevalence of over weight and obesity in different fat and sugar consumption Groups. (Abstract only) *Proceedings of the Nutrition Society* **52**, 383 A.

Cousins, J.H., Rubovitz, D.S., Dunn, J.K. *et al*. (1992) Family vs. individually oriented interventions for weight loss in Mexican American women. *Public Health Report* **7** (5), 549–555.

Department of Health Social Security Committee on Medical Aspects of Food Policy. (1987*)* *The use of very low calorie diets in obesity. Report on Health Social Subjects*. HMSO. London.

Formiguera, X. (1999) Diet in obesity management: appraisal and recommendations. In: *Obesity: The Threat Ahead*. p. 22. European Congress on Obesity.

Friedman, X. & Brownell, X. (1996) Chapter 11. In: *Hersen Sourcebook of Psychological Treatment Manuals for Adult Disorders*. (ed. Van Hesselt).

Frost, G. *et al*. (1991) A new method of energy prescription to improve weight loss. *Journal of Human Nutrition Dietetics* **4**, 369–373.

Garrow, J.S. (1992) Treatment of obesity. *Lancet* **30**, 409–413.

Henbest, R.J. & Stewart, M. (1990) Patient centredness in the consultation: does it really make a difference? *Family Practice* **7** (1), 28–33.

James, W.P.T., Schofield, E.C. & Jequier, E. (1994) Carbohyrdates as a sources of energy. *American Journal of Clinical Nutrition* **59**, 6825–6855.

Kushner, R. (1999) Integrated weight management approach. In: *Obesity. The Threat Ahead*, p. 36.

Lean, M.E.J. & James, W.P.T. (1986) Prescription of diabetic diets in the 1980s. *Lancet* **I**, 723–725.

Peabody, F.W. (1927) The care of the patient. *Journal of the American Medical Association* **88**, 877.

Prentice, A.M. & Jebb, S.A. (1995) Obesity in Britain: gluttony or sloth? *British Medical Journal* **311**, 437–439.

Sarvis, W.H.M. (1998) Physical activity in the treatment of obesity. *Symposium on Obesity – The Threat Ahead*. 24–25.

Shah, M. & McGovern, P., French S. *et al*. (1994) Comparison of a low fat – ad libetum complex carbohydrate diet with a low energy diet in moderately obese women. *Annals of Journal of Clinical Nutrition* **59**, 980–984.

8 Drug treatment in the management of obesity

INTRODUCTION

Controls over body weight, appetite and energy expenditure are both physiologically and voluntarily controlled and have evolved to protect against starvation. Therefore, it should not be surprising to clinicians that such mechanisms are not adapted to modern times when over-nutrition rather than under-nutrition is the major problem in the developed world.

Given these facts, it should not be surprising that dietary advice and voluntary control often fail to counteract basic physiological mechanisms and environmental factors.

Surely then it is legitimate to consider pharmacological treatments to reinforce dietary and lifestyle advice in certain categories of patients who are at high risk of premature death or major disability from their obesity and related risk factors or comorbid conditions.

In Chapter 5, the case was advanced for considering obesity as a disease in its own right; arguing that it should be accorded the status of a major chronic condition and managed accordingly.

In many ways its management can be likened to that of type 2 diabetes—one of its many consequences—the first stage is to advise dietary modification associated with an increase in physical activity. However, when these measures do not achieve metabolic control of the diabetic state, there is normally a willingness to resort to drug therapy to prevent, minimize or delay the complications of type 2 diabetes and thereby improve the quality of life.

Given the impact of obesity on both mortality and morbidity as outlined in Chapter 5, surely it is time to acknowledge that drug treatment has a part to play in weight loss and weight maintenance programmes in selected groups of patients. The guidance from the Royal College of Physicians (RCP 1998) is both welcome and timely and should stimulate clinicians to re-examine their attitudes to the use of drugs in managing these obese patients.

As Kopelman said (Kopelman 1998), 'antiobesity drugs should be considered as legitimate treatment for a serious medical disorder and not regarded as a panacea for moderate degrees of excess body fat'. WHO in classifying obesity as a disease recognizes that the use of drugs is an appropriate part of an overall management plan, which has to take a long-term perspective.

The ideal drug for the treatment of obesity would produce a dose-related weight loss, permit the user to achieve and maintain ideal body weight, be safe when used over long periods and have no tolerance or addictive potential (Jung 1997).

Unfortunately such a drug does not exist at the present time but research offers hope for the future.

The fact that the ideal drug for the treatment of hypertension or diabetes does not exist has not prevented us from using what is available to secure maximum benefits for patients. Treating such conditions almost always commits a patient to a lifetime of drug therapy but this does not always result in optimal control of either blood pressure in hypertensive people or the metabolic state in people with type 2 diabetes. Failure to secure the desired outcomes does not lead the clinician to abandon treatment but to review compliance and if necessary to consider alternatives.

Some years ago there was an understandable and wholly justified rejection of the use of drugs in managing obesity largely on the grounds of their addictive potential or ineffectiveness and poor tolerability. However, given the impact of obesity on both mortality and morbidity and the fact that newer non-addictive drugs are emerging, a re-examination of the place of drug therapy in its management is justified.

As mentioned in Chapter 3, with advancing years there is an aggregated fall in physical activity. The US Ageing Study (McGandy *et al.* 1966) suggested this could be 350 kcal/day in men (equates to four extra digestive biscuits per day). There is also an age related fall in basal metabolic rate (BMR) amounting to 40 kcal/day in men and 30 kcal/day in women between the ages of 25 and 75 years. Taken together these figures mean a decrease in energy expenditure of 700–800 kcal/day. Is it reasonable to assume that the appetite control system can cope with these changes in energy expenditure?

PRINCIPLES OF DRUG THERAPY IN OBESITY

Drug therapy should only be taken under strict medical supervision. It must be complementary to calorie restriction and increased physical activity, both of which must be maintained after drug therapy has been started. Drug therapy should be used for specific medical indications and not to improve appearance. A decision to start drug treatment should be based on the physician's judgement about the risks to an individual from continuing obesity.

- Drug treatment should not be considered ineffective because weight loss stops provided a 5–10% weight loss is achieved and maintained (RCP 1998).
- Drug treatment should be non-addictive and improve comorbid risk factors.
- Drug treatment should demonstrate a benefit that is greater than that achievable by dietary modification and increased physical activity alone.

- Weight loss on drug treatment should exceed that on placebo by at least 5% (Finer 1997). (However, weight loss in diabetics is difficult to achieve and any weight loss is beneficial.)
- Long-term use could be considered where multiple risk factors are present and considerable benefits are likely to result from weight loss not achievable by lifestyle modification alone.

SELECTION OF PATIENTS (BASED ON RCP 1998)

The following groups are suggested but clinicians will have to make individual choices and take account of factors such as age, family history, overall risk profile and the presence of other comorbid conditions.

- Patients with a BMI > 30 kg/m^2, with a strong family history of type 2 diabetes and premature coronary heart disease in a first degree relative who fail to achieve a 10% weight loss with lifestyle modification over a period of 3 months.
- Patients with a BMI > 28 kg/m^2 and with co-morbid conditions who fail to achieve a 10% weight loss after 3 months of supervised care.

In the opinion of the clinician, the patient's family history and personal risk profile justify seeking a 10% weight loss that has not been achieved by lifestyle changes alone.

CHOICE OF DRUG

Drugs such as the amphetamines, thyroxine and diuretics should never be used for weight reduction and dexfenfluramine has now been withdrawn. This effectively leaves the clinician with two drugs, orlistat and sibutramine.

Orlistat

This is a novel drug for the treatment of obesity in conjunction with a mildly hypocaloric diet in patients with a BMI > 30 kg/m^2 or BMI > 28 kg/m^2 with associated risk factors. The drug is supported by a comprehensive weight management programme. The Medical Action Plan (MAP) support line, manned by independent health care professionals, provides encouragement, motivational support and dietary advice to complement advice provided in the surgery.

Treatment should only be started if dietary modification and increased physical activity has produced a weight loss greater than 2.5 kg over 4 weeks and should be discontinued if treatment has not resulted in at least a 5% weight loss after 12 weeks.

A 16.4% weight loss can be achieved after 1 year when Xenical is prescribed according to license. This is associated with reductions of 10.6 mmHg of systolic and 8.4 mmHg in diastolic blood pressure; a reduction of 13.7% in LDL-cholesterol (Study 14119C data presented by Sjöström at ECO in Sjöström et al. 1998).

Mode of action

Orlistat inhibits the action of pancreatic lipase in the process of digesting fat so that approximately 30% of dietary fat is unabsorbed and subsequently excreted from the body, thereby reducing the amount of energy available to the body.

In clinical trials patients receiving orlistat lost almost twice as much weight as patients on a placebo and importantly in long-term trials designed to assess weight maintenance, patients on orlistat regained less weight than those on placebo.

Results of trials

In a 2-year randomized placebo controlled trial of orlistat, for weight loss and prevention of weight gain (Sjöström *et al.* 1998) the orlistat group lost; on average, more body weight than the placebo group (10.2% [10.3 kg]) vs. 6.1% [6.1 kg] at the end of year one. During year two, patients who continued orlistat regained on average half as much weight as those switched to placebo. Patients switched from placebo to orlistat lost an additional 0.9 kg in year two. In addition total cholesterol, LDL cholesterol LDL/HDL ratio and concentrations of glucose and insulin, decreased more in the orlistat group. However, gastrointestinal side-effects, the result of excretion of unabsorbed fat were more common in this group.

A randomized double-blind trial of long-term treatment of obesity in primary care settings (Hauptman *et al.* 2000) involving 17 primary care centres in the USA and 796 obese patients/BMI 30–44 kg/m². Patients were treated with placebo, 60 mg orlistat, or 120 mg orlistat, three times daily in three separate cohorts. Patients treated with orlistat lost significantly more weight than those treated with placebo and sustained more of their weight loss during year two. Also, orlistat produced greater improvements than placebo in serum lipid levels and blood pressure, and treatment was well tolerated. The researchers concluded that orlistat was an effective adjunct to dietary intervention in the treatment of obesity in primary care settings.

In a 2-year study on weight loss, weight maintenance and cardiovascular risk (Rossner *et al.* 2000) it was found that orlistat, administered for 2 years promotes weight loss and minimizes weight gain. Additionally, it led to significant improvements in lipid profile, blood pressure and quality of life. This was a multicentre, randomized double-blind, placebo controlled study. Overweight and obese patients (BMI 28–43 kg/m²) were randomized to placebo or orlistat 60–120 mg three times a day. Changes in body weight, lipid profile, blood pressure and quality of life, safety and tolerability were measured. Orlistat patients lost significantly more weight ($P < 0.001$) than placebo treated patients after year one (6.6%, 8.1% and 9.7% for the placebo, and orlistat 60 mg and 120 mg groups, respectively).

During the second year orlistat therapy produced less weight gain than placebo: ($P = 0.005$ for orlistat 60 mg; $P=0.001$ for orlistat 120 mg). Side-effects were predictable because of the mode of action of orlistat, but were generally mild and transient.

The 2-year studies with orlistat were designed to demonstrate weight loss in the first year, when all patients were encouraged to take a hypocaloric diet. **During the second year, which was designed to demonstrate weight maintenance, patients were advised to eat a eucaloric diet.**

A total of 3132 patients (BMI 28 43 kg/m^2) were evaluated in an analysis of pooled data from five randomized double-blind, placebo controlled trials of orlistat in conjunction with a hypocaloric diet (Zavoral 1998).

After one year, orlistat 120 mg produced significantly more weight loss than placebo (9.2% vs. 5.8%; $P > 0.01$).

A greater proportion of orlistat treated patients lost > 5% or > 10% of their initial body weight, compared to placebo (69.6% vs. 51.9% $P > 0.001$ and 42.1% vs. 22.7%; $P > 0.001$), respectively. Orlistat treated patients had significantly greater improvements than placebo treated patients in total cholesterol, LDL cholesterol, triglycerides and apolipoprotein B. In addition, orlistat had a beneficial effect on oral glucose tolerance, lipid status, waist circumference and systolic and diastolic blood pressure. Orlistat was well tolerated and had a similar safety profile to placebo.

A British one year randomized, double-blind study (Finer *et al.* 2000) concluded that orlistat, in conjunction with a low energy diet, produced greater and more frequent significant weight loss than placebo. One-third achieved clinically relevant weight loss (> 5% initial body weight). There was also improvement in relevant lipid parameters

In another randomized controlled trial using orlistat over a 2-year period (Davidson *et al.* 1999) it was found that treatment with orlistat promoted weight loss, lessened weight regain and improved obesity related risk factors. This involved 1187 subjects, 892 were randomly assigned on day one to double-blind treatment. During the first year orlistat-treated patients lost more weight (mean + SEM 8.76 + 0.37 kg) than placebo-treated subjects (5.81 + 0.67 kg) ($P < 0.001$). Also subjects treated with orlistat 120 mg, three times daily, regained less weight during year 2 (3.2 + 0.45 kg; 35.2% regain) than both those treated with orlistat 60 mg (4.26 = + 0.57 kg 51.3% regain) and placebo (5.63 + 0.42 kg, 63.4% regain). Treatment with orlistat was also associated with improvements in fasting LDL cholesterol and insulin levels.

Following the completion of pharmacokinetic interaction studies 'no interactions with biguanides, fibrates, digoxin, phenytoin, oral contraceptives, slow release nifedipine, nifedipine GITS or alcohol have been observed'. This is especially important for the concurrent use of orlistat and metformin in people with diabetes.

Orlistat, weight loss and diabetic control

In the Swedish multimorbidity study (Lingärde et al. 2000) a total of 382 obese adults (BMI 28–32 kg/m^2) with type 2 diabetes, hyperchols-terolaemia and/or hypertension were recruited, of whom 376 were ran-domized to orlistat (n = 190) or placebo (n = 186). After one year's treatment the mean weight loss was significantly greater with orlistat compared with placebo (5.9% vs. 4.6%; P<0.05). Moreover, signifi-cantly more orlistat-treated patients than placebo recipients maintained weight loss of at least 5% (54.2% vs. 40.9%; P < 0.001). Orlistat was also associated with significantly greater improvements than placebo in total cholesterol (– 7% vs. 1.1% P < 0.01) and HbAIC (– 2.7% vs. 0.5%; P < 0.05). It was also well tolerated.

Heymsfield (Heymsfield et al. 2000) reported a study on the use of orlistat and resultant weight loss on the progression to type 2 diabetes in obese adults, and found that the addition of orlistat to a convention-al weight loss regimen, significantly improved oral glucose tolerance, and diminished the rate of progression to the development of impaired glucose tolerance and type 2 diabetes.

In a randomized placebo controlled study of orlistat in overweight patients with type 2 diabetes treated with insulin (Kelley 2000) it was found that after 1 year, mean weight loss was significantly greater with orlistat than control (3.9% vs. 1.3% P = 0.0002). In addition more patients in the orlistat group than in the control group achieved a weight loss of > 5% (33% vs. 13%; P = 0.0001) or > 10% (10% vs. 4% P +0.0012). Treatment with orlistat resulted in significantly greater mean improvements in both HbAIC (– 0.62% vs. 0.27%; P +0.0021) and plasma glucose (– 1.63 vs. 1.08 mmol/L; P = 0.0219) compared with control. In addition, compared with control, significantly more patients in the orlistat group were able to reduce or discontinue the antidiabetic medication while fewer needed increased or additional medication (P < 0.001).

The links between visceral fat, insulin resistance and chronic cardio-vascular risk are well documented. It is of importance then to note that treatment with orlistat resulted in a reduced visceral fat area. A study by Mendoza-Guadaramma et al. reported a 16% reduction in visceral fat area in orlistat treated patients compared with only 2.4% for placebo (Mendoza-Guadaramma et al. 2000).

A study by Wilding (Wilding 1999) showed that treatment with orli-stat was accompanied by greater weight loss and improvements in insulin resistance (measured by the HOMA-R technique) than placebo. Greater weight loss with orlistat was maintained after 2 years treatment.

Weight loss in patients with type 2 diabetes is known to be accompa-nied by improved metabolic control and reduced cardiovascular risk factors. However, weight loss is notoriously difficult to achieve.

The results of a multi-centre, randomized double-blind, placebo con-trolled 57 week study (Hollander et al. 1998) are particularly important.

After one year of treatment the orlistat group lost $6.2 \pm 0.45\%$ of total body weight vs. $4.3 \pm 0.49\%$ in the placebo group ($P < 0.01$).

Twice as many patients in the treated group (49 vs. 23%) lost $\geq 5\%$ total body weight ($P < 0.001$).

Orlistat treated patients showed:

- Decreases in HbAIC ($P < 0.001$).
- Improvements in fasting plasma glucose ($P < 0.001$).
- Dosage reductions in sulphonylurea ($P < 0.01$).
- Reductions in total cholesterol ($P < 0.001$).
- Reductions in LDL cholesterol ($P < 0.001$).
- Reductions in triglycerides ($P < 0.05$).
- Reductions in Apolipoprotein B ($P < 0.001$) and
- Reductions in LDL to HDL ratio ($P < 0.001$). Only mild to moderate gastro-intestinal side effects were reported and vitamin supplementation was required in only a few patients (Hollander *et al.* 1998).

Orlistat, free fatty acids and insulin resistance of obesity

A study of the impact of orlistat treatment three times daily (Vidgren *et al.* 1999) showed that there was a significant decrease in the proportion of linoleic acid in triglycerides, cholesterol esters and phospholipids in the orlistat group compared with the placebo group, even after the effect of the decrease in dietary linoleic acid, weight change and gender were taken into account (Vidgren *et al.* 1999).

Orlistat has been shown to improve insulin sensitivity as measured by the euglycemic–hyperinsulinanemia glucose clamp (MCR) after three months treatment independently of any weight loss (Dahl *et al.* 2000).

Also combined orlistat and a hypocaloric diet improve insulin sensitivity more than diet alone (Özor *et al.* 2001).

Orlistat has been shown to promote weight loss, decrease insulin resistance and improve cardiovascular risk profile in obese patients with type 2 diabetes (Dimitror *et al.* 2001).

Orlistat has been shown to improve glycaemic control, lipid profile and blood pressure in obese patients treated with Metformin for type 2 diabetes. (Miles 2000).

Orlistat can be combined with Metformin for the treatment of type 2 diabetes. Metformin is of course the drug of choice for obese people with type 2 diabetes. A study (Miles *et al.* 2001) lasting one year which was randomized, double-blind and placebo controlled, multicentre yielded the following results. After one year weight loss was significantly greater in the orlistat group. A greater proportion of orlistat treated patients achieved 5% weight loss (39.0% vs. 15.7%; $P < 0.001$) and 10% weight loss (14.1% vs. 3.9%; $P < 0.001$). More orlistat treated patients had a decrease in HbAIC of 0.5% (61% vs. 43%; $P < 0.01$) and 1% (46% vs. 29%; $P < 0.01$). More patients in the treated group decreased or discontinued one anti-diabetic medication (17% vs. 8%). Fewer treated patients increased their anti-diabetic medication (12% vs. 22%) compared with placebo treated patients and the orlistat treated group had greater decreases in fasting glucose, total cholesterol LDL cholesterol, LDL/HDL ratio and systolic blood pressure. This data demonstrates that orlistat is a useful drug in obese type 2 diabetic patients.

Contra-indications

Contra-indications for orlistat are:
- Chronic malabsorption syndrome.
- Cholestasis.
- Breast feeding and known hypersensitivity to any component of the product. It is not recommended during pregnancy.

Adverse effects

The potential drawbacks to the drug are largely gastrointestinal and stem directly from its effect of inhibiting lipase. They are:
- Spotting from the rectum.
- Increased flatus with discharge.
- Fatty, oily stools.
- Faecal urgency.
- Increased defaecation.
- Possibly faecal incontinence.
- Bloating and abdominal discomfort.

All of the above tended to decrease with prolonged use and are less likely to occur when the patient adheres to appropriate dietary advice. In this respect orlistat almost has a 'antabuse effect' in encouraging dietary compliance. There is some evidence that these can be reduced by the use of a high fibre diet.

Precautions

Treatment with orlistat could potentially impair the absorption of fat soluble vitamins (A, D, E and K) although clinically important manifestations of this have not been reported so far. No clinical manifestations have been reported after 3 years' widespread use. It is highly important that patients are advised to comply with their dietary advice so as to minimize the risk of experiencing gastrointestinal side-effects.

Anti-diabetic drug treatment should be carefully monitored when patients are also taking orlistat as improvement in glycaemic control may warrant reduction in the dosage of anti-diabetic therapy.

Drug interactions

Long-term co-administration with warfarin should be closely monitored using INR values.

Dosage and administration

Adults should take one capsule (120 mg orlistat) immediately before, during or up to 1 hour after each main meal containing fat. Doses above 120 mg do not bring additional benefits. The daily intake of protein, fat and carbohydrate should be distributed over the three main meals and the diet should be mildly hypocaloric (30% of calories from fat).

It does appear that orlistat provides a new option for treating patients whose obesity puts them at significant risk but only as part of a weight loss and weight maintenance programme delivered under close medical supervision. At present there is no information about the efficacy and safety of orlistat beyond 2 years.

NICE recommendations: guidance on orlistat

1   Orlistat should only be prescribed for people who have lost at least 2.5 kg in weight by dietary control and increased physical activity alone in the month prior to the first preparation and meet one of the following criteria:

2   A body mass index (BMI) of 28 kg/m^2 or more in the presence of significant comorbidities which persist despite standard treatment (e.g. type 2 diabetes, high blood pressure and/or high total cholesterol level).

3   A BMI of 30 kg/m^2 or more with no associated comorbidities.

4   Orlistat should only be prescribed for people between the ages of 18 and 75 years.

5   When treatment with orlistat is offered, arrangements should be made for appropriate health professionals to offer specific concomitant advice, support and counselling on diet, physical activity and behavioural strategies.

6   Continuation of this therapy beyond 3 months should be supported by evidence of a loss of at least a further 5% of body weight from the start of drug treatment.

7   Continuation of this therapy beyond 6 months should be supported by evidence of cumulative weight loss of at least 10% of body weight from the start of drug treatment.

8   Treatment should not usually be continued beyond 12 months, and never beyond 24 months.

9   A patient support programme is available and funded by the manufacturers with a view to easing the role of primary care teams.

Sibutramine

Sibutramine offers three types of benefit in weight management:

(i)   Enhances weight loss.

(ii) Improves weight maintenance.

(iii) Reduces comorbidities.

A patient support programme is available funded by the manufacturers. Studies have shown that sibutramine, together with a life-style diet and exercise programme can achieve a clinically significant weight loss in about two-thirds of patients treated with the drug. Furthermore there is good evidence that the efficacy of the drug is maintained for up to 2 years with beneficial improvements in the traditional cardiovascular risk factors of the HDL cholesterol, LDL cholesterol and triglycerides. If these changes are put into equations that allow prediction of cardiac disease the results are, to say the least, encouraging (Dr N Finer, ECO Conference 2001).

Mode of action

Sibutramine has two complimentary physiological effects. First, it promotes and prolongs satiety after eating thereby reducing food intake, including snack consumption. Secondly, it stimulates energy expenditure and limits the decline in metabolic rate that normally accompanies weight loss (Stock 1997).

It has a twofold pharmacological action in that it is a monoamine re-uptake inhibitor, and is particularly effective in blocking the re-uptake of both seratonin and noradrenaline. In this respect it is different from drugs such as dexfenfluramine which act by stimulating the release of monoamines. Sibutramine is not associated with the risk of primary pulmonary hypertension and possible heart valve incompetence seen with dexfenfluramine nor does it have mood altering and addictive effects.

Results of trials

It is important to recognize that treatment with sibutramine is in addition to dietary advice and increased physical activity and in no way replaces either.

All trial data has included appropriate lifestyle modification.

In obese individuals sibutramine causes a dose related weight loss (Weintraub *et al.* 1991), and in a 12-week trial:

- 5 mg per day resulted in a 2.9-kg weight loss.
- 20 mg per day produced a 5.0-kg weight loss.
- Placebo led to a 1.4-kg weight loss.

    (Licensed doses of sibutramine are 10 mg and 15 mg).

    In a study of 485 patients in 12 UK general practices (Jones & Heath 1996), out of the 225 patients who completed 12 months' treatment, the following weight losses were achieved:

- 8.3 kg on placebo.
- 10.2 kg on 10 mg daily of sibutramine.
- 10.5 kg on 15 mg of sibutramine.

    Further important findings are that 5% loss of body weight was achieved by 20% of those on placebo, by 40% of those on sibutramine 10 mg daily, and in 57% by those on 15 mg sibutramine daily.

    Sibutramine resulted in a dose related weight loss over a range of 5–30 mg per day and this weight loss can be maintained for 12 months, if the non-responders—about 10% of patients—are withdrawn because they have failed to lose 1% of their body weight. The remaining 90%

can be expected to lose 7.7 kg and maintain this weight loss over 12 months provided that they heed dietary advice and take increased exercise (Lean 1997).

Evidence is accumulating that the weight loss achieved by treatment with sibutramine is associated with improvements in glucose homeostasis and improved blood pressure control.

In a trial using sibutramine as an aid to weight loss in obese patients with type 2 diabetes it was found that:

Sibutramine did not prevent the improvement in insulin sensitivity associated with weight loss. Patients treated with sibutramine showed a significant reduction in weight loss when compared to the placebo group.

The relationship between dose and weight loss was reported in March 1999 (Bray *et al.* 1999). Seven clinical centres screened 1463 patients who were then randomized to 24-week treatment with one of six doses of sibutramine or placebo. The respective doses of sibutramine were 1, 5, 10 and 15, 20 or 30 mg once daily. Six hundred and eighty-three patients completed the study and a 2-week placebo run-in period was used to initiate a standardized programme of weight loss involving dietary modification, physical activity and lifestyle changes.

For those completing the 24-week trial the results were as follows:

Placebo	1.2%
1 mg	2.7%
5 mg	3.9%
10 mg	6.1%
15 mg	7.4%
20 mg	8.8%
30 mg	9.4%

Weight loss was dose related and statistically significant vs. placebo (p < 0.05) for doses of 5 mg and upwards.

Furthermore weight loss achieved at 4 weeks was predictive of weight loss at 24 weeks.

Patients losing weight also showed:

- Increase in high density lipoprotein (HDL).
- Reduction in serum triglycerides.
- Low density lipoprotein (LDL) and uric acid.

There were small mean increases in blood pressure and pulse rate and the most frequently reported adverse events were dry mouth, anorexia and insomnia all of which are related to the pharmacology of sibutramine.

A 3-month multicentre, placebo controlled study (Barbe *et al.* 1999) reported at the European Congress on Obesity, sibutramine 15 mg was compared with placebo on body composition changes following weight loss in obese patients. Ninety-two patients were screened and 83 were randomized to sibutramine (43) and placebo (40). There were five withdrawals from the sibutramine group and six from placebo.

There was a 7.9 kg weight loss in the sibutramine group compared with 3.3 kg in the placebo arm of the trial. This weight loss was associated with favourable changes in the body composition in sibutramine treated patients compared to placebo particularly in reduction in the visceral fat mass reflected in observed reductions of weight circumference (7.6 cm compared with 4.0 cm).

Although there have been many other trials assessing the effectiveness of sibutramine in weight loss and weight management programmes, by far the most important is the Sibutramine Trial in Obesity Reduction and Maintenance (STORM); preliminary data from which was released at the European Congress on Obesity held in Milan in June 1999.

STORM results

Storm Trial (James *et al.* 2000). This involved 605 obese patients (BMI 30–46kg/m^2) for a six month period of weight loss with sibutramine (10mgs/day) and an individualized 600kcal/day deficit programme based on measured resting metabolic rates.

The 467 (77%) patients who achieved 5% weight loss were then randomly assigned to sibutramine 10mgs/day (*n* = 352) or placebo (*n* = 115) for a further 18 months.

Sibutramine was increased to 20mgs/day if weight gain recurred.

148 (42%) individuals in the sibutramine group and 58 (50%) in the placebo group dropped out. Of the 204 sibutramine treated individuals who completed the trial 89 (43%) maintained 80% or more of their weight loss, compared with 9 (16%) of the 57 individuals in the placebo group.

Patients had substantial decreases over the first six months in respect of triglycerides, VLDL cholesterol, C peptide and uric acid which were sustained in the treated but not in the placebo group.

HDL cholesterol concentrations rose substantially in the second year with overall increases of 20.7% in the sibutramine group and 11.7% in the placebo group. Twenty patients (3%) were withdrawn because blood pressure became elevated. The mean increase in blood pressure in the study population was by 0.1 mmHg (SD12.9), diastolic blood pressure by 2.3 mmHg (9.4) and pulse rate by 4.1 beats/min (11.9).

The individualized management programme achieved weight loss in 77% of obese patients and sustained weight loss in most patients continuing treatment for two years.

Changes in HDL cholesterol, VLDL cholesterol and triglyceride but not LDL concentrations exceeded those expected from weight loss alone or when induced by other selective treatments for low concentrations of HDL cholesterol (James *et al.* 2000).

Sibutramine, weight loss and diabetic control

A randomized placebo controlled, double-blind, parallel group, 12 week study was conducted at two hospital based obesity/diabetes clinics. (Finer *et al.* 2000). The patients were men and women aged 30–65 years, with a BMI > 26 kg/m^2 and < 35 kg/m^2 and treated or untreated type 2 diabetes, diagnosed more than 6 months previously. Each patient was given sibutramine 15 mg or placebo once daily, and advised to follow a customized diet of 500 kcal/day less than the individual's energy needs. Ninety-one patients were randomized into the study; 44 to placebo and 47 to sibutramine 15 mg once daily. Eighty-three patients (91%) completed the study, 40 (91%) on placebo and 43 (91%) on sibutramine. The mean weight reduction from base line was statistically significantly greater with sibutramine than with placebo at every measurement and at the end of the study (2.4 vs. 0.1 kg at week 12; $P > 0.001$; intent to treat). The proportion of patients who lost more than 5% of their base line body weight was 19% in the sibutramine group and 0% in the placebo group ($P > 0.001$; 95% confidence interval: 9, 30). Patients receiving sibutramine lost significantly more fat mass compared with those receiving placebo, as a percentage (1% vs. 0.1%; $P > 0.05$) and in absolute terms (1.8 vs. 0.2 kg, $P > 0.001$). Loss of lean mass was not significantly different between the groups. Mean peak blood glucose concentration after a standard test meal decreased by 1.1 mmol/L in the sibutramine treatment group but increased by 0.5 mmol/L in the placebo group ($P = 0.04$; difference in means 1.6, 95% confidence interval: –3.3,—0.1). Mean fasting blood glucose decreased by 0.3 mmol/L with sibutramine and increased by 1.4 mmol/L with placebo. Mean glycosylated haemoglobin levels decreased by 0.3% with sibutramine treatment but were unchanged with placebo. Sibutramine 15 mg was deemed to be safe and well tolerated, and adverse events were mostly mild or moderate in severity. No significant differences were found between treatment groups in blood pressure, no clinically significant conduction or rhythm abnormalities were observed on ECG.

Sibutramine, free fatty acids and insulin resistance of obesity

The relationship between insulin mediated glucose disposal and day long free fatty acid (FFA) concentrations before and after sibutramine assisted weight loss was investigated in 24 healthy normotensive, non-diabetic obese women (BMI > 30kg/m^2) (McLaughlin 2001). The 24 volunteers were defined as being insulin resistant (IR) or insulin sensitive (IS) on the basis of their steady state plasma glucose (SSPG) concentration in response to 180 minute continuous intravenous infusion of octreotide, insulin and glucose. The main SSPG concentrations were significantly higher ($P > 0.001$) in the IR group (219 ± 7 vs. 69 ± 6 mg/dL) at base line. The IR group also had significantly higher plasma glucose ($P = 0.002$), insulin ($P > 0.01$), and SSA p = 0.02) concentrations measured at hourly intervals from 8 am to 4 pm before and after breakfast (ATM) and lunch (noon). Weight loss in response to an energy restricted diet for

4 months and sibutramine at 15 mg once daily was comparable in the two experimental groups (8.6 ± 1.3 vs. 7.9 ± 1.4 kg). SSPG concentrations decreased significantly ($P > 0.001$) following weight loss (219 ± 7–144 ± mg/dL) in the IR group. There was no change in the SSPG of the IS group (69 ± 6–73 ± 7 mg/dL). The improvement in insulin sensitivity in the IR group after weight loss was associated with a significant decline in day-long plasma glucose ($P > 0.001$) and insulin ($P = 0.02$) concentrations, without a weight loss associated decrease in day long plasma FFA responses. In contrast there was no significant change in plasma, glucose, insulin, and FFA concentrations following weight loss in the IS group. These results indicate that day-long FFA concentrations vary substantially in obese individuals as a function of whether they are IR or IS. Furthermore, the observation that the IR group was more IS after weight loss associated with lower day-long insulin concentrations in the absence of a significant decrease in circulating FFA concentrations suggests that resistance to insulin-mediated glucose disposal in obese individuals cannot be entirely due to high FFA levels.

Indications

Sibutramine is indicated for treatment of obese patients with a BMI > 30 kg/m^2 responding inadequately to non-pharmacological measures (less than 5% weight loss in 3 months) and for those who have a BMI > 27 kg/m^2 with comorbidities such as type 2 diabetes or dyslipidaemia.

Monitoring

Blood pressure and pulse rate should be monitored in all patients at least three times before the start of treatment, every second week in the first 3 months, monthly between 4 to 6 months, and regularly (at least every third month) after 6 months. Sibutramine should be discontinued if the rising heart rate increases by more than 10 beats per minute or if blood pressure increases by more than 10 mmHg at two consecutive visits.

Contra-indications

History of major eating disorders, psychiatric illness, Gilles de la Tourette syndrome, history of coronary heart disease, congestive heart failure, tachycardia, peripheral vascular disease, arrhythmias, cerebrovascular disease, uncontrolled hypertension, hyperthyroid disease, prostatic hypertrophy, phaeochromocytoma, angle closure glaucoma, history of drug or alcohol abuse, hepatic impairment, pregnancy and breast feeding.

Adverse effects

The side-effect profile of sibutramine is in keeping with its noradrenergic action. They include dry mouth, anorexia, constipation, insomnia, increased heart rate, palpitations, hypertension, vasodilation, lightheadedness, paraesthesia, headache, anxiety, sweating, taste disturbance, rarely blurred vision, but have only led to modest withdrawal of patients from trials—less than 1%.

Precautions

Monitor blood pressure and pulse rate (every 2 weeks for the first 3 months, monthly for 2 months then at least every 3 months thereafter)—discontinue if blood pressure or pulse rate elevated at two consecutive visits; sleep aponea syndrome; epilepsy; hepatic impairment (avoid if severe); renal impairment (avoid if severe); monitor for pulmonary hypertension (but effect not reported with sibutramine).

Duration of treatment—treatment should be discontinued if:

- Weight loss after 3 months less than 5% of initial body weight.
- Weight loss stabilises at less than 5% of initial body weight.
- Individuals regain 3 kg or more after previous weight loss.

In individuals with comorbid conditions, treatment should be continued only if weight loss is associated with other clinical benefits.

Drug interactions

- Antidepressants: increased risk of CNS toxicity (the manufacturer of sibutramine recommends avoiding comcomitant use); avoid sibutramine for 2 weeks after stopping MAOIs).
- Antipsychotics: increased risk of CNS toxicity (the manufacturers of sibutramine recommend avoiding comcomitant use).

There are possible interactions with dihydroergotamine, meperidine, phentayl, pentazocine, dextromethorphan (found in cough medicines), lithium, and tryptophan. Sibutramine may interact with ketoconazole, erythromycin, over-the-counter cough and cold medications, allergy medicines, and decongestants.

Dosage and administration

All patients should start with 10 mg of sibutramine once daily, thereafter the dose can be increased to 15 mg, if well tolerated, for patients losing less than 2 kg in the first month of treatment. Treatment should be discontinued if weight loss is inadequate, i.e less than 2 kg after 4 weeks of treatment. It should only be given in conjunction with a long-term programme consisting of diet, exercise and lifestyle modification. Sibutramine can be used for periods of up to 1 year but should be discontinued in patients whose weight loss stabilises at less than 5% of their initial body weight or who lose less than 5% of their initial body weight in 3 months on treatment or who regain more than 3 kg of an initial weight loss. Duration of treatment 1 year, **child, adolescent** under 18 years, and **elderly** over 65 years not recommended.

Taken orally in the morning.

NICE recommendations: guidance on sibutramine

1 Sibutramine should be prescribed only as part of an overall treatment plan for management of nutritional obesity in people aged 18–65 years who meet one of the following criteria:

   (a) A body mass index (BMI) of 27.0 kg/m^2 or more in the presence of significant comorbidities.

   (b) A BMI of 30.0 kg/m^2 or more without associated comorbidities.

2 Sibutramine should be prescribed, in accordance with the Summary of Product Characteristics, only for people who have made previous serious attempts to lose weight by diet, exercise and/or other behavioural modifications.

3 When treatment with sibutramine is offered, arrangements should be made for appropriate health professionals to offer specific concomitant advice, support and counselling on diet, physical activity and behavioural strategies. Sibutramine should not be prescribed unless adequate arrangements for monitoring both weight loss and adverse effects can be made available.

4 The starting dose of sibutramine should normally be 10 mg/day. Continuation of this therapy beyond 4 weeks should be supported by evidence of a 2 kg weight loss, and beyond 3 months should be supported by evidence of a loss of at least 5% of initial body weight from the start of drug treatment. Dosage may be increased to 15 mg/day after 4 weeks in line with sibutramine's Summary of Product Characteristics, and the same treatment and monitoring regimens followed as for the 10 mg/day dose. Sibutramine therapy should be stopped if there is inadequate response, as defined above.

5 Since the use of sibutramine may increase blood pressure of some individuals, blood pressure must be checked regularly in all those to whom it is prescribed. If blood pressure increases, continuation of sibutramine therapy must be reconsidered taking into account the risks and benefits of the effects of treatment on cardiovascular risk profile for the individual. Treatment with sibutramine is not recommended for individuals whose blood pressure before start of therapy is above 145/90 mmHg. Treatment should be discontinued in people whose blood pressure rises above 145/90 mmHg or by more than 10 mmHg (systolic or diastolic) or whose resting pulse rate rises by more than 10 beats per minute.

6 Treatment is not recommended beyond the licensed indication of 12 months.

7 There is no evidence to support the co-prescribing of sibutramine with other pharmacotherapy aimed at weight reduction.

THE FUTURE

Orlistat and sibutramine are imperfect but nonetheless valuable additions to the armamentarium of the clinician faced with trying to combat the impact on health of the burgeoning epidemic of obesity.

Bray (Bray 1998b) has provided an overview of the many different mechanisms that can be called on to alter the storage of body fat and its distribution. Basically new drugs can:

- Reduce food intake.
- Block food absorption.
- Reduce gastric emptying.
- Stimulate thermogenesis.
- Influence fat or protein metabolism of storage.
- Moderate the central controller.

In many ways the drug treatment of obesity today is analogous to the drug treatment of hypertension in 1958. Bray (1998a) has compared the arrival of orlistat for the former to the introduction of chlorotithiazide for the latter—one produces the loss of calories in the form of undigested triglycerides, the other the loss of sodium in a diuresis. He says, 'If today for obesity is analogous to 1958 for hypertension, then we can expect a variety of new and effective drugs'. Treating obesity effectively, like treating hypertension effectively could involve influencing a combination of the above mechanisms.

REFERENCES

Barbe, P.L., Hanotin, C. & Louvet, F.P. (1999) Effects of Sibutramine on the Body Composition Following Weight Loss in Obese Patients.

Bray, G. (1998a) Current and contemporary management of obesity. *Handbook on Healthcare.* New Town, PA.

Bray, G.A. (1998b) Strategies for discovering drugs to treat obesity. In: *Clinical Obesity* (eds P.G. Kopelman & M.J. Stock), pp. 508–544. Blackwell Science, Oxford.

Bray, G.A., Blackburn, G.L., Ferguson, J.M. *et al.* (1999) Sibutramine produces dose related weight loss. *Obesity Research* **7** (99), 189–198.

Dahl, D.B., Bachman, O.P., Brechtel, K. *et al.* (2000) Effects of orlistat on insulin sensitivity (IS) in obese intentionally weight maintaining subjects. Abstract 600, European Association Study of Obesity (EA50).

Davidson, M.H. *et al.* (1999) Weight control and risk factor reduction in obese weight control and risk factor reduction in obese subjects treated for two years with orlistat. *JAMA* **281**(3), 235–242.

Dimitror, D., Koeva, L., Kovatchera, T. *et al.* (2000) Effect of Orlistat on insulin resistance, cardiovascular risk factors and serum leptin levels in obese type 2 diabetic patients. *International Journal of Obesity* **24** (Suppl 1).

Finer, N. (1997) Present and future pharmacological approaches. *British Medical Bulletin* **53**, 409–432.

Finer, N. & Bloom, S.R. (2000) Sibutramine is effective for weight loss and diabetic control in obesity with type 2 diabetes: a randomised, double blind, placebo controlled study. *Diabetes, Obesity and Metabolism* **2** (2), 105–112.

Finer, N., James, W.P.T., Kopelman, P.G. *et al.* (2000) One year treatment of obesity: a randomised, double blind, placebo controlled, multicentre study of orlistat, a gastrointestinal lipase inhibitor. *International Journal of Obesity* **24**, 306–313.

Hauptman, J. *et al.* (2000) Orlistat in the long-term treatment of obesity in primary care settings. *Archives of Family Medicine* **9**, 160–167.

Heymsfield, S.B., Segal, K.R., Hauptman, J. *et al.* (2000) Effects of weight loss with orlistat on glucose tolerance and progression to Type 2 diabetes in obese adults. *Archives of International Medicine* **160**, 1321–1326.

Hollander, P.A., Elbein, S.C., Hirsch, I.B. *et al.* (1998) Role of orlistat in the treatment of obese patients with Type 2 diabetes. *Diabetes Care* **21** (8), 1288–1294.

James, W.P.T., Astrup, A., Finer, N. *et al.* (2000) Effect of sibutramine on weight maintenance after weight loss: a randomized trial. *Lancet* **356**, 2119–2125.

Jones, S.P., Heath, M.J. (1996) Long term weight loss with sibutramine; 5% responders. *International Journal of Obesity* **20** (Suppl. 4), 157. Abstract.

Jung, R.T. (1997) Obesity as a disease. British Medical Bulletin **53**, 307–321.

Kelley, D. (2000) Effect of orlistat in overweight Type 2 diabetic patients receiving insulin. Manage Weight-Manage Type 2 diabetes: New Orlistat Data. *Roche Satellite Symposium. 17th International Diabetes Federation Congress, Mexico City.*

Kopelman, P. (1998) Antiobesity drugs. *Family Medicine* **2**, 28.

Lean, M.E.J. (1997) Sibutramine—a review of clinical efficiency. *International Journal of Obesity* **21**, 530–536.

Lingärde, F. *et al.* (2000) The effect of orlistat on body weight and coronary heart disease risk profile in obese patients. The Swedish Multimorbidity Study. *Journal of International Medicine* **248**, 245–254.

McGandy, R.B., Barrows, C.H. Jr, Spanias, A. *et al.* (1966) Nutrient intake and energy expenditure in men of different ages. *Journal of Gerontology* **21**, 581–587.

McLaughlin, T., Abbasi, F., Lamendola, C. *et al.* (2001) Metabolic changes following sibutramine-assisted weight loss in obese individuals: role of plasma free fatty acids in the insulin resistance of obesity. *Metabolism* **50**, 819–824.

Mendoza-Guadaramma, L.G., Lopez-Alvarenga, J.C., Castillo-Martinez. (2000) Orlistat reduces visceral fat independent of weight changes in obese type 2 diabetes. *International Journal of Obesity* **24**(Suppl. 1), 5167. Abstract.

Miles, J.M. (2000) Role of orlistat in overweight metformin-treated patients with Type 2 diabetes. Manage Weight-Manage Type 2 diabetes: New Orlistat Data. *Roche Satellite Symposium. 17th International Diabetes Federation Congress, Mexico City.*

Miles, J.M., Aionne, L., Hollander, P. *et al.* (2001) Effects of orlistat in overweight and obese type 2 diabetic patients treated with metformin. *Diabetologia* **44** (Suppl 13), 1–12. Abstract 890, EASO.

Özer, E.M., Ayter, M., Güren, D. (2001) Effect of weight reduction in insulin resistance and glucose tolerance with orlistat treatment in obese patients. Abstract 692, EA50 2001.

Rossner, S. *et al.* (2000) Weight loss, weight maintenance, and improved cardiovascular risk factors after 2 years treatment with Orlistat for obesity. *Obesity Research* **8**(1), 49–61.

Royal College of Physicians. (1998) *Clinical Management of Overweight and Obese Patients with Particular Reference to the Use of Drugs.* RCP, London.

Sjöström, L., Rissanen, A., Anderson, T. *et al* (1998) Randomised placebo-controlled trial of Orlistat for weight loss and prevention of weight regain in obese patients. *Lancet* **352**, 167–173.

Stock, M.J. (1997) Sibutramine: a review of the pharmacology of a novel antiobesity agent. *International Journal of Obesity* **21** (Suppl.), 1525–1529.

Vidgren, H.M., Agren, J.J., Valere, R.S. *et al.* (1999) Clinical *Pharmacology and Therapeutics* **66**, 315–322.

Weintraub, M., Rubio, A., Golik, X *et al.* (1991) Sibutramine in weight control: a dose ranging, efficacy study. Clinical *Pharmacology and Therapeutics* **50,** 330–337.

Wilding, J. (1999) Orlistat induced weight loss improves insulin resistance of serum lipid fractions in obese subjects. *Diabetalogica* **42** (Suppl.), Abstract 215.

Zavoral, J.H. (1998) Treatment with Orlistat reduces cardiovascular risk in obese patients. *Journal of Hypertension* **16**, 2013–2017.

9 The place of surgery in the management of obesity

INTRODUCTION

In the previous chapter on the place of drug therapy in the management of obesity, a case was advanced for the use of drug therapy in a selected group of patients.

To take this argument a stage further is to recognize that on occasions lifestyle advice supported by drug treatment does not achieve the desired results and, as a result, some patients remain at considerable risk of premature death or significant disability. For such patients surgery provides an option worth considering as surgical treatments do have evidence of success in achieving and maintaining medically significant weight loss over meaningful periods of time (Kral 1998).

The WHO in recognizing obesity as a disease, acknowledges that surgery should be considered in the management of its more extreme forms but only as part of a comprehensive weight management plan.

While most patients with obesity are treated with lifestyle advice and in some cases with drugs, for those with morbid obesity (body mass index (BMI) >40) such an approach is unlikely to deal adequately with their problems.

If left untreated patients who are morbidly obese (1–2% of the population) in the UK have only a one in seven chance of achieving their normal life expectancy.

In the last decade the National Institutes for Health in the US and the Scottish Intercollegiate Guidelines have suggested that surgery is the most effective treatment for selected patients with morbid obesity and both organizations have recommended that surgery be carried out more frequently.

In 1991 a survey in the UK showed that there were only 38 obesity surgeons and a repeat survey in 1998 showed that the number had dropped to 23.

It is little wonder that the UK is so far behind Europe the US and Australia in effectively tacking a major health problem.

SELECTION OF PATIENTS

The selection criteria for surgery have been defined by the International Federation for the Surgery of Obesity:

- BMI > 40 or 35–40 in patients with serious comorbidities treatable by weight loss.

- Being obese for a minimum 5 years.
- Failure of conservation treatment.
- Aged between 18 and 55 years.
- Acceptable operative risk.

   Data from the Scottish obese subjects study (Nashund & Agten 1999) showed that surgery is overwhelmingly better than conservative treatment in:

- Improving quality of life.
- Curing type 2 diabetes.
- Controlling hypertension.
- Reducing atheroma.
- Improving rates of employment.
- Reducing healthcare costs.

   Other studies (Kral 1995) have also shown improvements in:

- Lipid profiles.
- Sleep apnoea.
- Musculoskeletal problems.
- Oesophageal reflux.
- Urinary incontinence.
- Asthma.

   Sadly, society and the medical profession are too often ignorant and prejudiced against the morbidly obese and fail to recognize that obesity needs to be treated just like any other serious disease.

   The results of surgery are impressive. Data from over 14 000 patients on the International Register of Obesity Surgery shows that at 12 months vertical banded gastroplasty and gastric bypass result in a mean loss of 53 and 72% of excess weight, respectively, with an operative mortality of only 0.17% (Mason *et al.* 1997), 93% of patients have no morbidity.

   Laparoscopic insertion of a gastric band resulted in patients losing 50–60 lb of their excess weight and maintaining this for at least 6 years (Belachew *et al.* 1998).

   It has to be borne in mind that the safety of surgical procedures has improved considerably with the introduction of minimally invasive techniques and in addition, costs of treatment have to be taken into consideration. A comparative study in the US (Martin *et al.* 1995) concluded that the cost for each kilogram of weight lost was less for surgical than medical treatment when looked at over a 5-year period.

PROCEDURES

   In the UK surgical treatment has been centred on achieving either gastric restriction by creating a smaller capacity stomach or on creating a state of malabsorption by intestinal bypass (jejuno-ileal) surgery.

   The latter method carries with it a very high rate of complications both in the immediate post-operative period and in the medium and long-term (NIH 1991) to the extent that the Scottish Intercollegiate Guidelines Network (SIC 1996) advised against its use in the management of obesity. The same organization came down in favour of gastric plication as the preferred operation arguing that very substantial improvements in the morbidity of patients with extreme BMIs occur after this operation (NIH 1991; Brolin *et al.* 1994).

SIDE-EFFECTS

The commonest side-effect after gastric bypass is vomiting. Most often this is from a failure of the patient to adapt eating behaviour to the reduced capacity of the stomach but it can be indicative of the development of a stricture requiring endoscopic dilatation.

As with peptic ulcer surgery, gastric bypass can result in dumping syndrome with a prevalence of between 20 and 70% (Van der Kleij 1996) and this can be improved by dietary counselling.

COMPLICATIONS

These include the development of anaemia which can be related to B_{12} deficiency (loss of intrinsic factor) or to iron deficiency.

A comprehensive list of side-effects and complications is shown in Fig. 9.1 below:

These are formidable lists and reinforce the message that surgery is only justified in the management of obesity when other measures have failed to produce the desired results and the patients risk profile justifies radical action.

RESULTS

Surgical procedures to combat obesity have been shown to improve most comorbid conditions.

Fig 9.1 Possible side-effects and complications of gastric bypass surgery.

Side-effects	Complications
Dumping 70%	Vitamin B_{12} deficiency 25%
Constipation 40%	Incisional hernia 15%
Intolerance to dairy products 50%	Vomiting 15%
Headache 40%	Iron deficiency anaemia 15%
Hair loss 33%	General vitamin deficiency (not B_{12}) 10%
Depression 15%	

Type 2 diabetes

In a study comparing 154 patients with type 2 diabetes who had undergone gastric bypass with 72 type 2 patients who had elected against surgery there was a fivefold reduction in mortality (MacDonald *et al.* 1997). In a series of 100 patients (Pories *et al.* 1995) gastric bypass was shown to prevent the progression of glucose intolerance to frank type 2 diabetes.

Syndrome X

Anti-obesity surgery has been shown to improve hypertension (Carson *et al.* 1994) and hyperlipidaemia (Barakat *et al.* 1992) so that is likely to delay or prevent the progression of Syndrome X to premature cardiovascular disease and possibly death.

Cancer

It has been suggested that anti-obesity surgery can play a part in preventing obesity-related cancers such as breast (Schapira *et al.* 1994) prostate and colon. So far there is a lack of sound epidemiological data to substantiate this claim.

Safety laparoscopic procedures performed in specialist centres carry a lower mortality than actuarial mortality in the severely obese.

References

Barakat, H.A., McLendon, V.D., Marks, R. *et al.* (1992) Influence of morbid obesity and non insulin dependant diabetes mellitus on high density lipoprotein composition and subpopulation distribution. *Metabolism* **41**, 37–41.

Belachew, H., Legnand, M., Vincent, V. *et al.* (1998) Laparoscopic adjustable gastric banding. *Werla Geurnel Surgery* **22**, 955–963.

Brolin, R.E., Robertson, L.B., Kewler, H.A. *et al.* (1994) Weight loss and dietary intakes after vertical banded gastroplasty and Roux-en-Y gastric bypass. *Annals of Surgery* **220**, 782–790.

Carson, J.L., Ruddy, M.E., Duff, A.E. *et al.* (1994) The effect of gastric bypass surgery on hypertension in morbidly obese patients. *Archives of Internal Medicine* **154**, 193–200.

Kral, J.G. (1995) Obesity. In: Lubin, M.F. *et al.* (eds) *Medcial Management of the Surgery Patient*, 3rd edn. Lipincott, Philadelphia P.A. pp.415–423.

Kral, J.G. (1998) Surgical treatment of obesity. In: Eds Kopelman P.G., Stock, M.J. *Clinical Obesity*. Blackwell Science, Oxford pp.545–563.

MacDonald, K.G., Long, S.D., Swanson, M.S. *et al.* (1997) The gastric bypass operation reduces the progression and mortality of non insulin dependent diabetes mellitus. *Journal of Gastrointestinal Surgery* **1**, 213–220.

Martin, L.F., Tan, T.L., Horn, J.R. *et al.* (1995) Comparison of the costs associated with medical and surgical treatment of obesity. *Surgery* **118**, 599–607.

Mason, E.E., Tang, S., Renquiat, K.E. *et al.* (1997) Decade of change in obesity surgery. *Obesity Surgery* **7**, 189–197.

Nashund, I. & Agten, G. (1999) Is obesity surgery worthwhile? *Obesity Surgery* **9**, 36.

National Institutes for Health Consensus. (1996) Statement. Gastrointestinal surgery for severe obesity. *Nutrition* **12**, 379–340.

NIH Consensus Development Conference Panel. (1991) Gastro-intestinal surgery for severe obesity. *Annals of Internal Medicine* **115**, 956–961.

Pories, W.G., Swanson, M.S., MacDonald, K.G. *et al.* (1995) Who would have thought it? An operation proves to be the most effective treatment for adult onset diabetes mellitus. *Annals of Surgery* **22**, 339–352.

Schapira, D.V., Clark, R.A., Wolff, P.A. (1994) Visceral obesity and breast cancer risk. *Cancer* **74**, 632–639.

Scottish Intercollegiate Guidelines Network. (1996) Obesity in Scotland. Integrating prevention with weight management. *Scottish Intercollagate Guidelines Network*.

Shiffman, M.L., Sugerman, H.J., Kellum, J.M. *et al.* (1994) Gallstone formation after rapid weight loss: a prospective study in patients undergoing gastric bypass surgery for treatment of morbid obesity. *American Journal of Gastroenterology* **86**, 1000–1005.

van der Kleij, F.G., Vecht, J., Lamers, C.B. *et al.* (1996) Diagnostic value of dumping provocation in patients after gastric surgery. *Scandinavian Journal of Gastroenterology* **31**, 1162–1166.

10 The economic consequences of obesity

INTRODUCTION

The economic costs of obesity in the developed world are considerable. There are the direct costs of diagnosis, treatment, and management of diseases associated with obesity, and the indirect costs which reflect the loss of productivity due to obesity.

The costs in some westernized countries are discussed below. These refer mainly to the direct costs with the exception of the USA.

UNITED KINGDOM

Direct costs of treating obesity are shown in Fig. 10.1.

Fig 10.1 Direct costs of treating obesity and its consequences.

	Cost £ million
General practitioner consultations	6.8
Admissions	1.3
Prescriptions	0.8
Out patient attendances	0.5
Day cases	0.1
Total costs	9.5

Treating the consequences of obesity

Prescriptions	247.2
Admissions	120.7
Out patient attendances	51.9
General practitioner consultations	44.9
Day cases	5.2
Total costs of treating consequences of obesity	469.9
Total direct costs	479.4

Source: National Audit Office estimates

Indirect costs

These are defined in terms of lost output due to sickness or death and were estimated to be in the region of £2.1 billion in England in 1998, of which £1.3 billion was due to sickness absence caused by obesity and £0.8 billion due to premature mortality (National Audit Office 2001).

These are clearly not representative of current expenditure since the prevalence of obesity is increasing along with increasing numbers of older people in the population. They do, however, indicate that health care costs associated with obesity are considerable and likely to escalate.

Fig 10.2 Costs of overweight and obesity as a risk factor for other diseases.

Disease	Date	Total Cost £mm	% due to obesity	Obesity est. £mm
Myocardial infarction	1990	155	5	7.75
Stroke	1985	550	5	27.5
Type 2 diabetes	1986/7	484	80	100
Osteoarthritis	1989	495	10	30
Hypertension		N/A	20	N/A
Total		**1684**		**165.25**

Source: Office Health Economics

UNITED STATES

Work by Colditz (Colditz 1992) using a prevalence-based approach estimated that the costs accountable to obesity in 1986 were $39.3 billion. He included direct and indirect costs in reaching this figure and pointed out that it might in fact be too low because cancers and musculoskeletal disorders were not included.

Obesity accounted for:

- 57% of the costs of type 2 diabetes;
- 19% of the costs of cardiovascular disease;
- 26% of the costs of hypertension.

The figure of $39.3 billion was calculated to represent 5.5% of the total costs of illness.

FRANCE

Using a cut-off point of 27 kg/m^2 the proportion of diseases accountable to obesity were 25% for hypertension and stroke, and 3% for breast cancer. The direct costs of obesity were estimated to be about 2% of the cost of the French health system (Levy *et al.* 1995).

AUSTRALIA

Estimates of the medical costs of obesity (BMI $\geq$30 kg/m^2) amounted to 4% of pharmaceutical expenditure, 2% of the costs of medical consultations and 16% of recurrent hospital expenditure (Segal *et al.* 1994).

FINLAND

The National Survey on Health and Social Security revealed that the costs of medication increased by about 120% when the BMI increased from 25 to 40 kg/m^2.

In a Finnish study (Rissanen *et al.* 1990) obesity was associated with a twofold increased risk of premature disability in men and a 1.5-fold greater risk in women.

SWEDEN

The SOS Study (Sjöström *et al.* 1995) is a nation-wide intervention which is showing major reductions in obesity related diseases after surgically induced weight loss. The reduction in the incidence of diabetes was 17-fold and there were 3–23-fold decreases in the 2 years' incidence of cardiovascular diseases.

The data available suggests that about 4–8% of healthcare expenditure is attributable to obesity. This does not take into account the indirect costs such as loss of productivity due to premature death and disability, which are likely to be in excess of the direct costs. Studies in Sweden of women aged 30–59 years (Narbro *et al.* 1996) showed that approximately 10% of the total cost of the loss of productivity due to sick leave and disability pensions was thought to be related to obesity and its associated conditions.

THE FUTURE

The future in terms of healthcare expenditure is bleak, as the prevalence of obesity is rising and the population are living longer. Yet the benefits of a 5–15% weight loss are considerable in improving the health of individuals and reducing both the direct and indirect healthcare costs associated with obesity, so that much greater attention to both its prevention and treatment would seem to be justified.

References

Colditz, G. (1992) Economic costs of obesity. *Annals of Clinical Nutrition* **55**, 5035–5075.

Levy, E., Levy, P., Lepen, C. *et al.* (1995) The economic costs of obesity: the French situation. *International Journal of Obesity* **19**, 790–792.

Narbro, K., Jonsson, E., Larsson, B. *et al.* (1996) Economic consequences of sick leave and early retirement in obese Swedish women. *International Journal of Obesity* **20**, 895–903.

National Audit Office. (2001) *Tackling Obesity in England*. The Stationery Office, London.

OPCS (1990). When weight gets out of control. In: *Doctor 1992*. The Office of Population, Censuses and Surveys. pp. 48–49.

Rissanen, A., Heliovaara, M., Knekt, P. *et al.* (1990) Risk of disability and mortality due to overweight in a Finnish population. *British Medical Journal* **301**, 835–837.

Segal, C.L., Contre, R. & Zimmet, P. (1994) The cost of obesity: the Australian perspective. *Pharmacoeconomics* **5** (Suppl. 1), 45–52.

Sjöström, L., Narbro, K. & Sjostrom, D. (1995) Costs and benefits when treating obesity. *International Journal of Obesity* **19** (Suppl. 6), S9–S12.

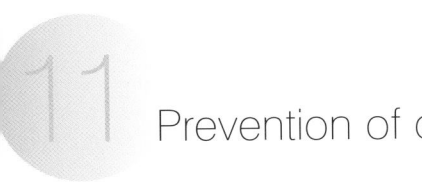

Prevention of obesity

INTRODUCTION

If people could be persuaded and helped to avoid becoming obese it would bring enormous benefits to individuals in terms of improved quality of life and longevity as well as significant savings in health and expenditure.

Individuals would benefit from a reduced likelihood of developing type 2 diabetes, cardiovascular disease, osteoarthritis and certain cancers and the National Health Service would be relieved of the costs of treating them.

Reasons for preventing obesity

- Obesity is a chronic condition which is often recalcitrant to treatment.
- Obesity is associated with a wide range of debilitating conditions; imposes a huge burden on healthcare costs and deserves recognition as an important disease entirely in its own right.
- The prevention of obesity should figure more prominently in Health Improvement Programmes as it has such an important role in the development of type 2 diabetes, ischaemic heart disease, certain cancers and a range of other important medical conditions.

TWO APPROACHES

Two major approaches are possible (Rose 1986):

- the population based; and
- the personal high risk.

The former attempts to reduce the prevalence of obesity across whole communities while the latter targets high-risk individuals.

The two approaches are entirely complimentary and the reality is that both will be required if we are to control the epidemic of obesity in the western world.

The major interventions that have been proposed are:

- Increasing the level of physical activity especially in those with very sedentary lifestyles.
- Reducing the saturated fat content of the diet with a compensatory increase in the intake of complex carbohydrates and fruit and vegetables.

It is worth emphasizing that the target is the prevention or reduction in the prevalence of those conditions associated with obesity not the achievement of 'ideal' bodyweight.

The population approach

There is much to be learned from the population based programmes aimed at the primary prevention of coronary heart disease—the North Karelia Project (Puska *et al.* 1985) and in California the Stamford Four Communities Study (Farquhar *et al.* 1990).

While these studies demonstrated a reduction of saturated fat intake, smoking habits, serum cholesterol and blood pressure, they did not demonstrate significant reductions of obesity. This is probably because it is difficult (outside of wartime) to influence the food supply of populations. To do this, it would be necessary to co-ordinate agricultural production, food manufacturing processes and marketing practices in a way which influences consumer choice for the better. In other words, agricultural, economic and health policies must be integrated if we are to achieve the desired changes. This is, of course, a major challenge to government and one which it is hoped will be tackled by the Food Standards Agency.

The emergence of Health Action Zones provides an opportunity to deliver community based weight management programmes, in collaboration with the local food industry, local leisure facilities, health education departments, and co-ordinated by public health physicians.

The high risk approach

This is particularly suited to the British system of primary care. About 75% of the population see their general practitioner in one year (RCGP 1994) and approximately 90% over a five-year period. The average number of contacts between the average patient and the average NHS general practitioner has been rising in recent years and is now as high as five per year (OPCS 1991).

Thus the opportunities exist to identify opportunistically the high-risk patient and offer appropriate advice which could then be supplemented by support from community based clinics (see Organization of services, p. 49).

Advice on modification of diet and increased physical activity is largely as discussed in Chapter 7.

Groups that could be targeted

Suggested groups at which a preventive approach could be targeted are:
- Those with a family history of obesity and type 2 diabetes in a first degree relative.
- Those with a family history of obesity and a history of premature coronary heart disease in a first degree relative.
- Women entering pregnancy with a BMI $\geq 25\,\text{kg/m}^2.$
- Those giving up smoking.

RECOMMENDATIONS

Professor Philip James has produced a series of recommendations relating to active living, sport and leisure and diet which could well be the basis of any population based approach to the prevention of obesity. They are reproduced by kind permission of Professor James (James 1995).

Active living

Recommendations for active living (James 1995).

1 Long-term planning of town and city centres should encourage and sometimes require a progressive increase in walking and cycling.
2 Measures are needed to encourage walking and cycling as a means of travel for short journeys. The measures include:
   - Traffic speed limits.
   - Traffic calming.
   - Traffic banning in some areas.
   - Provision of safe footpaths and cycling routes.
   - Provision of safe cycle parking facilities.
   - Special measures to improve access to low cost reflective bands and cycle helmets.
   - Financial incentives for walking, cycling and public transport.
   - Disincentives for car use.

Sport and leisure activity

Recommendations for sport and leisure activity in the prevention of obesity (James 1995).

1 Targets for physical activity need to be defined for different groups of people which specify the time spent in different levels of activity.
2 Pre-school facilities should encourage active play.
3 Schools should emphasize the fun and health benefits of sport and leisure for all, and allow experience of a wide range of sports.
4 Schools should encourage activity outside school by:
   - Encouraging walking and cycling for leisure.
   - Provide links to clubs and community activities.
   - Re-evaluating the payment and hours of work of teachers involved in extra curricular sport.
5 Work places should encourage:
   - Awareness of health targets.
   - Sport/leisure participations by provision of facilities and opportunities.
   - Walking, cycling and public transport for work related journeys.
6 Local authorities should encourage access to leisure facilities and make special provision for:
   - Mothers, babies and small children.
   - Children and adolescents.

- The elderly.
- The unemployed.
- GP prescription referrals.
- Those who are unfit or overweight or unfamiliar with facilities: those groups who need a sympathized approach.

Dietary issues

Recommendations concerning dietary issues in the prevention of obesity (James 1995).

1 Concerted effort to reach the 30% fat target in the UK.
2 The fat content of food to be displayed in government, local authority and staff restaurants.
3 Targets to be displayed in public eating houses.
4 Accentuate the drive to reduce the fat content of food.
5 Nutritional information for customers to be developed in a more easily understood form with simple visual aids.
6 Standards set for nursery, school and hospital meals.
7 Schools should teach:
- Skills to use a wide range of foods.
- Healthy nutrition and active lifestyle across the curriculum and by example and practice.

References

Farquhar, J.W., Fortman, S.P., Flora, J.A. *et al.* (1990) Effect of community-wide education on cardiovascular risk factors; The Stanford Five-City Project. *Journal of the American Medical Association* **264**, 359–365.

James, W.P.T. (1995) A public health approach to the problem of obesity. *International Journal of Obesity* **19**(Suppl. 3), 537–545.

Office of Population Consensus and Surveys (1991).

Puska, P., Salonen, J. & Nissinen, A. (1983) Change in risk factors for coronary heart disease during 10 years of community intervention programme: North Karelia Project. *British Medical Journal* **287**, 1840–1844.

RCGP (1994) *Nutrition in General Practice 1: Basic Principles of Nutrition.* Royal College of General Practitioners, London.

Rose, G. (1986) Sick individuals and sick populations. *International Journal of Epidemiology* **14**, 32–38.

12 Childhood obesity

NORMAL DEVELOPMENT

In normal development BMI rises steeply in the first 12–18 months of life and this is followed by a gradual but sustained fall which levels off at about 6–7 years of age, after which there is a gradual increase over time (Davies 1994).

Children whose BMI rises earlier than normal tend to be those who become overweight or obese in childhood.

EPIDEMIOLOGY

The prevalence of obesity in childhood appears to be increasing.

In the USA the National Health Examination Surveys (NHES) and the National Health and Nutrition Examination Surveys (NHANES) have shown that since the early 1960s there has been:

- A 54% increase in the prevalence of obesity between 1963 and 1980 in children ages 6–11 years.
- A 98% increase in levels of super obesity (skin fold thickness greater than the 95th centile).
- Increases of a similar magnitude were seen in children aged 12–17 years. In England and Scotland broadly similar data were provided by the National Studies of Health & Growth in 1972, 1980 and 1990.

Other studies have shown that similar trends are occurring in Europe and the Middle East.

One recent study (Barth *et al.* 1997) shows that there has been a significant increase in the magnitude of obesity in obese children and adolescents.

Three independent cross-sectional surveys of children in England and Scotland using internationally agreed cut off points showed that there was little change in the prevalence of overweight and obesity between 1974 and 1984. However, from 1984 to 1994:

- Overweight increased from 5.4% to 9.0% in English boys and from 6.4% to 10% in Scottish boys.
- Overweight increased from 9.3% to 13.5% in English girls and 10.4% to 15.8% in Scottish girls.
- The prevalence of obesity reached 1.7% in English boys and 2.1% in Scottish boys and 2.6% in English girls.

These trends have serious implications for the prevalence of adult obesity (Chinn & Rona 2001).

However, in children aged 1.5–4.5 years the position is more stable. The National Diet and Nutrition Survey showed no significant difference in mean BMI compared with children in a 1968 survey (DHSS 1975).

In fact in some groups mean weight was lower than the 1968 levels in spite of these being a mean increase in stature of 3.5 cm over the same period.

Approximately 5% of children are overweight at the age of 7 years. It is more common in girls than boys and by the age of 9 years the figure has increased to 9% (Braddon et al. 1986). Garrow (1991) has proposed that there should be a policy of identifying overweight children in primary schools as he feels that the problem is best tackled between the ages of 7 and 11 years. This would require the close co-operation of parents, teachers, school nurses and community dieticians as well as the primary care team.

This suggests that the development of childhood obesity is predominantly a post 5 years of age problem.

LINKS BETWEEN CHILDHOOD AND ADULT OBESITY

The impact of obesity on health is detailed in Chapter 5. While childhood obesity is associated with short term largely psychological damage—poor self image, impaired peer relationships and family interactions (Sallade 1973)—the longer term impact on health when childhood obesity persists into adult life must not be lost sight of.

ASSESSMENT OF CHILDHOOD OBESITY

There are a number of methods which can be used to assess obesity in childhood, some are very expensive (dual X-ray absorptiometry) others that children find unpleasant (skinfold calipers). However, BMI is a fairly good index of body size and has been in use for many years. As BMI in childhood changes markedly with age, it has to be assessed by using age related references. These are now available (Cole et al. 1995).

GROWTH CHARTS

Growth charts for boys and girls which incorporate BMI are essential for assessing obesity in children. They are available from the Child Growth Foundation 1996/1 (Charity Registration Number 274325, 2 Mayfield Avenue, London W4 1PW) and include advice on referral (examples are shown in Appendix 2).

AETIOLOGY OF CHILDHOOD OBESITY

While genetic factors certainly play a part, they can hardly be held responsible for the increasing prevalence outlined previously. As Prentice and Jebb (Prentice & Jebb 1995) have pointed out this burgeoning of obesity has occurred against a background of a relatively constant gene pool so that environmental and behavioural influences must have played the major role (see also Chapter 3).

Changes in the composition of the diet with increase in the fat content are probably more important than the total energy content which appears to be decreasing.

Perhaps of even greater importance is the evidence that total energy expenditure has declined markedly over the past 30 years.

Studies in three different centres, Phoenix (USA), Berlington (USA) and Cambridge (UK) all produced remarkably similar results (Davies *et al.* 1991, 1994; Fontvieille *et al.* 1993; Goran *et al.* 1993):

- Phoenix Study 24% below current recommendations.
- Burlington Study 23% below current recommendations.
- Cambridge Study 15–25% below current recommendations.

These findings are undoubtedly a major contributory factor in the development of the escalating problem of childhood obesity.

MANAGEMENT

Any attempt to normalize a child's weight should be done in the context of the family unit and not in isolation. The giving of dietary advice should be through a dietician as there is the need to carefully consider the nutrient quality of the diet in children who are still growing.

The use of medication is not licensed in children so the only possible methods are dietary change and increased physical activity.

Dietary change

Any dietary intervention to reduce calorie intake must take into account the essential need to provide through the diet the essential micronutrients such as calcium and iron.

Probably the simplest approach is to limit the intake of dietary fat because:

- The energy density of fat means that it is easy to consume large quantities of calories quickly.
- Fat is less satiating than carbohydrate.
- Fat does not stimulate thermogenesis in the way that carbohydrate does.
  Another approach is the so called traffic light diet (Epstein *et al.* 1990). In this approach foods are colour coded:
- red—energy dense—to be used sparingly;

- amber—moderately energy dense—to be used in moderation;
- green—low energy dense—to make up the bulk of the diet.

Physical activity

Any programme to increase physical activity should be combined with dietary intervention.

Any exercise programme should be carefully designed and monitored and should:

- Take into account the maturity of the child.
- Take account of the fact that children are more susceptible than adults to heat injury.
- Be 'fun' to aid compliance.
- Be capable of being home based and not require special equipment or clothing.

In designing programmes of dietary intervention and physical activity, it is imperative to aim for long-term compliance and not short-term gain. There is an advantage in treating obesity in childhood in that children 'grow into their weight'—their height will increase for a number of years so that if weight can be kept stable BMI will improve.

Obesity and the ages of man (Rossiter 2001).

Life period	Thrust of intervention
Prenatal	Prevention
Childhood and adolescence	Prevention and treatment
Young adults	Treatment and prevention
Middle age	Treatment
Elderly	Selective treatment.

References

Barth, N., Zeigler, A., Himmelman, G.W. *et al.* (1997) Significant weight gains in a clinical sample of obese children and adolescents between 1985 and 1995. *International Journal of Obesity* **21**, 122–126.

Braddon, R.E.M *et al.* (1986) Onset of obesity in a 36 year birth cohort study. *British Medical Journal* **293**, 259–303.

Chinn, S. & Rona, R.J. (2001) Prevalence and trends in over weight and obesity in three cross-sectioned studies of British children, 1974–94. *British Medical Journal* **322**, 24–26.

Cole, T.J., Freeman, J.V. & Price, M.A. (1995) Body mass index reference curves for the UK, 1990. *Archives of Disease of Childhood* **73**, 25–29.

Davies, P.S.W., Coward, W.A., Gregory, J. *et al.* (1994) Total energy expenditure and energy intake in the pre-school child: a comparison. *British Journal of Nutrition* **72**, 13–20.

Davies, P.S.W., Livingstone, M.B.E., Prentice, A.M. *et al.* (1991) Total energy expenditure during childhood and adolescence. *Proceedings of the Nutrition Society* **50**, 14a.

DHSS. (1975*) Report on Health Social Subjects: 10. Nutrition Survey of Pre-School Children 1967–68.* Department of Health and Social Security: London. HMSO.

Epstein, L.H., Valoski, A., Wing, R.R. *et al.* (1990) Ten year follow-up of behavioural family based treatment for obese children. *Journal of American Dietetics Association* **264**, 2519–2523.

Fontvieille, A.M., Harpor, I.T., Ferraro, R.I. *et al.* (1993) Daily energy expenditure by five-year-old children, measured by doubly labelled water. *Journal of Paediatrics* **123**, 200–207.

Garrow, J.S. (1991) Importance of obesity. *British Medical Journal* **303**, 704–706.

Goran, M.J., Carpenter, W.H. & Poehlam, E.T. (1993) Total energy expenditure in 4–6 year-old children. *American Journal of Physiology* **264**, E706–E711.

Prentice, A.M. & Jebb, S.A. (1995) Obesity in Britain: gluttony or sloth? *British Medical Journal* **311**, 437–439.

Sallade, J. (1993) A comparison of the psychological adjustment of obese and non obese children. *Journal of Psychosomatic Research* **17**, 89–96.

a¹ Healthy eating

In 1990 the Government published '*Eight Guidelines for a Healthy Diet*' (MAFF/DoH/HEA, 1990). The guidelines are produced here with added comments from the RCGP Nutrition Working Party (RCGP 1994):

1 Enjoy your food.

2 Eat a variety of foods (see Fig. A1).

3 Eat the right amount to be a healthy weight (as was indicated in Chapter 1).

The prevalence of overweight and obesity in Britain is increasing.

Fig A.1 The balance of good health. Based on Health Education Authority recommendation.

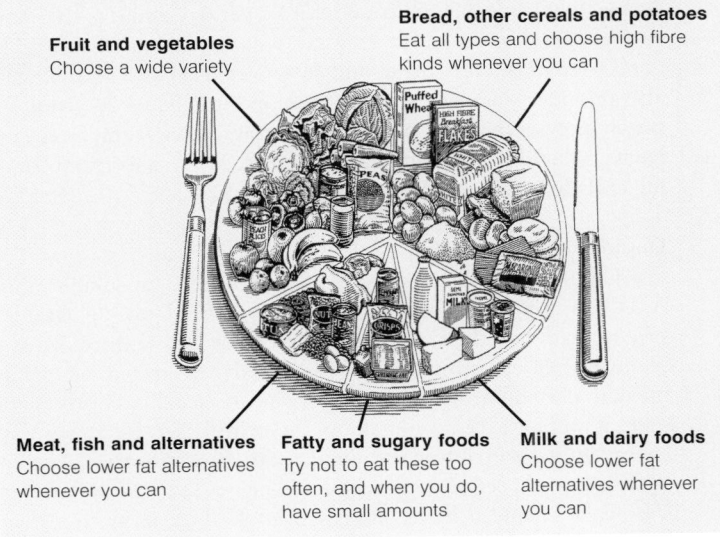

Fruit and vegetables
Choose a wide variety

Bread, other cereals and potatoes
Eat all types and choose high fibre kinds whenever you can

Meat, fish and alternatives
Choose lower fat alternatives whenever you can

Fatty and sugary foods
Try not to eat these too often, and when you do, have small amounts

Milk and dairy foods
Choose lower fat alternatives whenever you can

Most people if they eat to appetite are able to maintain a stable body weight over a period of time, i.e. they eat what they need; but it must be remembered that even 102% of energy intake above expenditure can, over a period of time, result in considerable weight gain and there has been a general decline in physical activity within increasing dependence on motorized transport.

The normal physiological response to reduced energy requirements is to down regulate appetite. However, this physiological response has to contend with the social convention of eating food because it is offered rather than needed. This makes it increasingly difficult to control energy intake, so that any advice on diet should always be coupled with advice on taking more exercise. A reduction in the level of obesity is one of the diet and nutrition targets contained in the Health of the Nation Report (Secretary of State for Health 1992).

4 Eat plenty of foods rich in starch and fibre.

Starch which is a form of carbohydrate is found in large amounts of cereals and root vegetables (see Fig. A1) and these foods should form a basis of most meals because they are filling without being too fattening. The Report on Dietary Reference Values (DoH, 1991) suggests that on average about 40% of the calories we eat should come from starch and intrinsic milk sugars. Another advantage of starchy foods is that they are usually rich in fibre (non-starch polysaccharides, NSP). Non-starchy polysaccharides help to prevent constipation. The average intake of NSP in Britain is 12 g per day and it is recommended that this is increased to 18 g per day for adults. As well as being good sources of fibre, bread and cereals are rich in B vitamins. Bread also provides some calcium and iron and it is better to acquire non-starch polysaccharides from foods rather than from bran supplements, which in large amounts may reduce the absorption of some minerals from other foods.

5 Do not eat too much fat.

Some fat in the diet is essential to provide the fat soluble vitamins A, D, E and K. Small amounts of fat make food more palatable and give many foods their characteristic flavour and texture. Most people in Britain eat too much fat, particularly saturated fat. Although the actual amount of fat that we eat has been falling in recent years there is still an excessive intake in the British diet. By eating less fat, energy intake will automatically be reduced. Although this is helpful for those who need to lose weight, in general reductions in fat intake should be balanced by an increased intake of starchy foods rich in fibre and by eating plenty of fruit and vegetables.

6 Do not eat sugary foods too often.

Eating less sugar is a good way to cut down energy intake for those who need to lose weight and sugar is also the main cause of tooth decay, particularly if it is taken in the form of sweet drinks and snacks. Sugar eating as part of a meal is less likely to cause tooth decay because it is washed away with other food and drink. The Coma Report (DoH, 1989) particularly identified non-milk extrinsic sugars as the likely cause of dental caries. Extrinsic sugar is not found within the cellular structure of foods, examples include sucrose, honey, glucose, glucose syrups and the sugar which occurs in fruit juices and other drinks. Although the sugar in milk (lactose) is also extrinsic, the Coma Report regarded milk sugar as a special case as it is not harmful to teeth. The other categorization of sugars used by the Coma Report was intrinsic sugar, by those found within the cellular structure of some unprocessed foods, such as fruit and vegetables. It is recommended that there is a reduction in the intake of non-milk extrinsic sugar from a national average of 14% of food energy to 11% to hope lessen the prevalence of dental caries.

7 Look after the vitamins and minerals in your food.

Eating a good variety of foods and having a good intake of fruit and vegetables regularly is an important way in seeing that vitamin requirements are met.

8 If you drink do so within sensible limits.

Current recommendations are 21 units of alcohol per week for men and 14 units for women. Single units are as follows:

- Half pint of beer or lager.
- A glass of wine.
- A single measure of spirits.
- A small glass of sherry.
- One and a half pints of low alcohol beer.
- Three glasses of low alcohol wine.

References

Department of Health (1991) *The Report on Dietary Reference Values*. London HMSO.

Department of Health (1992) *Health of the Nation: a Strategy for Health in England*. London HMSO.

Ministry of Agriculture, Fisheries and Food, Department of Health and Health Education Authority (1990) *Eight Guidelines for a Healthy Diet*. London HMSO.

Royal College of General Practitioners (1994) *Nutrition in General Practice 1 Basic Principles of Nutrition*. RCGP London.

a² Characteristics of successful weight management programmes

In a Department of Health funded evaluation of weight management services published as a supplement to the *Journal of Human Nutrition and Dietetics* in April 1999 it was found that:

1 Successful sustained clinically significantly clinical weight reduction in obese patients is rare.

2 Successful weight loss is achieved through multicomponent schemes which bring about lifestyle changes to reduce energy intake *and* increase energy output in ways which are practical and easy to sustain.

3 Regular contact and supportive follow-up are important in achieving and sustaining weight loss.

The evaluation showed that:

- Health related anxiety is the most common and potent factor in initiating weight loss.
- An assessment of readiness for lifestyle change should precede enrolment in a weight loss programme.
- Patients must want to lose weight.
- Any depression should be treated before starting attempts at weight loss.
- Treatment packages should be individualized.
- Verbal recommendation to join weight loss programmes works best for women from ethnic minorities.
- High coronary heart disease (CHD) risk status is a powerful motivator.
- Aiming for 'ideal' weight is unrealistic.
- Regular follow-up is important.
- Group sessions are more likely to be successful.
- Dietary advice combined with exercise programmes works better than dietary advice alone.
- Dietary advice aimed at the whole family improves compliance.
- Increasing physical activity should be dependent on attendance at a facility.
- Aquafit sessions are acceptable for those with joint problems.
- Exercise needs a higher profile.
- Support for exercise programmes by GPs and health professionals is helpful.

- Obese patients prefer to exercise with other obese patients.
- Exercise schemes which encourage participation of friends or partners are welcomed.
- Including a clinical psychologist in the professional team helped with behaviour modification (Thomas 1999).

The above points are certainly worth considering when designing weight loss and weight maintenance programmes.

Reference

Hughes, J., Martin, S. (1999) The Department of Health Project to evaluate weight mangement services. *Journal of Human Nutrition and Dietetics* **12** (Suppl. 1). 1–8.

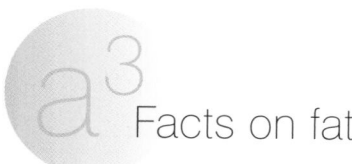

Facts on fat

Fat

Fat is the most concentrated available food source of energy.
There are three main types:

- Saturated fatty acids (saturates).
- Monounsaturated fatty acids (monounsaturates).
- Polyunsaturated fatty acids (polyunsaturates).

All foods contain a mixture of these fatty acids and it is an oversimplification to refer to a food as 'saturated' or 'unsaturated'. Butter contain 68% saturates, 23% monounsaturates and 4% polyunsaturates while the fatty acid profile of sunflower margarine is 17% saturates, 27% monounsaturates and 52% polyunsaturates.

Saturates

In saturates, the carbon atoms are fully saturated with hydrogen with the result that they are chemically very stable. Saturates are found mainly in foods of animal origin and in hard margarines (those have undergone a process of hydrogenization which converts unsaturates into saturates).

Other foods which contain saturates are biscuits, cakes and pies. Saturates tend to be solid at room temperature and high intakes both promote obesity and raise blood cholesterol—a major risk factor for developing coronary heart disease.

Monounsaturates

These contain a single unsaturated 'double bond' between two carbon atoms. Oils such as rape seed and olive oil are rich sources of monounsaturates.

Polyunsaturates

These contain between two and six double bonds which makes them much less chemically stable than saturates and much more liable to oxidation which is the process by which they become rancid. Unlike saturates they cannot be synthesized in the body. Several of the short chain fatty acids are deemed essential because they cannot be synthesized and therefore have to be provided in the diet. A moderate intake of polyunsaturates combined with a reduction in saturates tends to lower cholesterol and reduce the risk of heart disease. Sources of polyunsaturates are oily fish, mackerel, sardines, pilchards, salmon and green leafy vegetables.

Cholesterol

This is present in all foods of animal origin and is an essential component of every cell. The body synthesizes in the liver most of its requirements. It is a basic building block for the synthesis of steroid hormones, bile salts and vitamin D.

High intakes of saturates increase the liver synthesis of cholesterol and can lead to high levels of blood cholesterol and an increased risk of developing coronary heart disease.

Reference

RCGP (1994) *Nutrition in General Practice 1: Basic Principles of Nutrition.* RCGP, London.

a⁴ BMI charts

These are available from the Child Growth Foundation, who also supply the Cole Calculator which enables the height and weight for boys and girls to be used not only to calculate the current BMI, but also to relate this to the adult BMI. It is commended to the reader as an extremely useful and inexpensive piece of equipment.

© Child Growth Foundation.`

In Spring 2002 an updated version of the chart will be published featuring both the International Obesity Task Force (IOTF) cut-offs for overweight and obesity and the first waist centile charts standards to be published in the UK. If you would like to await publication before, register your interest by contacting Harlow Printing, Maxwell Street, South Shields NE33 4PU.

Referral guidelines

Refer a girl whose BMI falls above the 98th centile as obese. Consider referral, as overweight, a girl whose BMI falls above the 91st centile even on the basis of a single measurement. Consider for referral a girl whose BMI falls below the 2nd centile as being significantly underweight even on the basis of a single measurement. During infancy large but transient changes in centile may occur due to the shape of the charts, and these changes are normal. It should be remembered that the earlier the age of the second rise, the greater the risk of future obesity. Remember also that while BMI has a high correlation with relative fatness or leanness it is actually assessing the weight-to-height relationship: **this may give misleading results in girls who are very stocky and muscular who might appear obese on the BMI alone.**

GIRLS
BMI CHART
(BIRTH - 20 YEARS)
United Kingdom cross-sectional reference data : 1997/1

Name..

NHS No. ☐☐☐ ☐☐☐ ☐☐☐☐

How to calculate BMI

Divide weight (kg) by square of length/height (m²)
e.g. when weight = 25kg and length/height = 1.2m (120cm),
$$BMI = 25 \div (1.2 \times 1.2) = 17.4$$

Date	Age	Length/Height	Weight	BMI	Initials
: :	:	:	:	:	
: :	:	:	:	:	
: :	:	:	:	:	
: :	:	:	:	:	
: :	:	:	:	:	
: :	:	:	:	:	
: :	:	:	:	:	

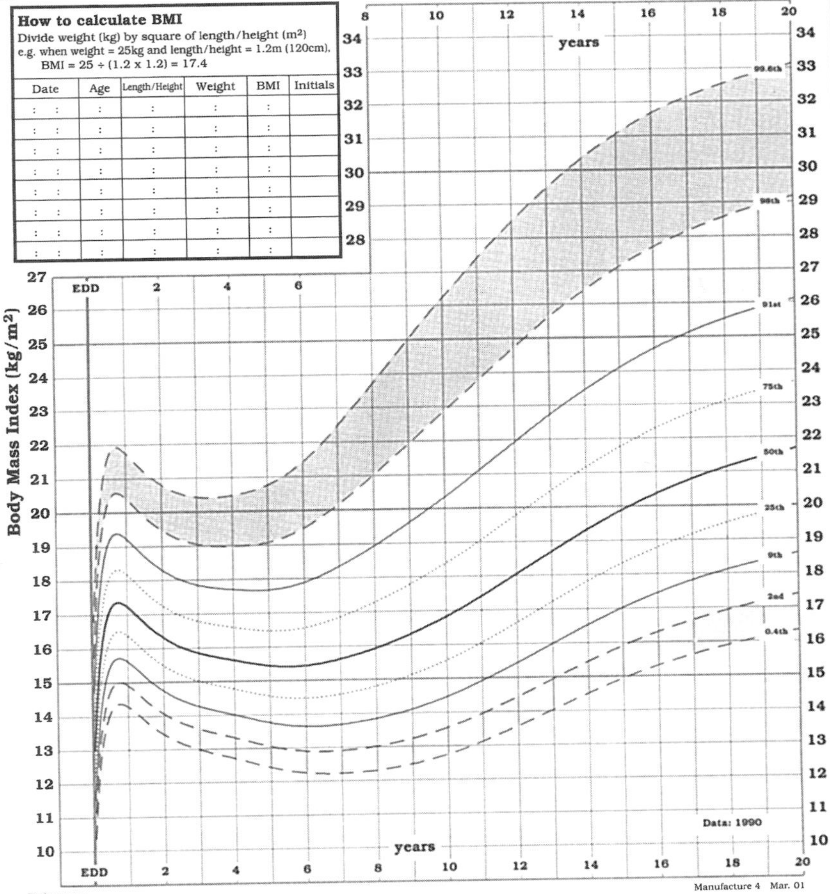

Body Mass Index (kg/m²)

Centile lines: 99.6th, 98th, 91st, 75th, 50th, 25th, 9th, 2nd, 0.4th

Data: 1990

Manufacture 4   Mar. 01

Reference

Body Mass Index reference curves for the UK, 1990 (TJ Cole, JV Freeman, MA Preece) *Arch Dis Child* 1995; **73**: 25-29
Sex differences in weight in infancy (MA Preece, JV Freeman, TJ Cole) *BMJ* 1996; **313**: 1486

Designed and Published by
© CHILD GROWTH FOUNDATION 1997/1
(Charity Reg. No 274325)
2 Mayfield Avenue,
London W4 1PW

Printed and Supplied by
HARLOW PRINTING LIMITED
Maxwell Street ◊ South Shields
Tyne & Wear ◊ NE33 4PU

Referral guidelines

Refer a boy whose BMI falls above the 98th centile as obese. Consider referral, as overweight, a boy whose BMI falls above the 91st centile even on the basis of a single measurement. Consider for referral a boy whose BMI falls below the 2nd centile as being significantly underweight even on the basis of a single measurement. During infancy large but transient changes in centile may occur due to the shape of the charts, and these changes are normal. It should be remembered that the earlier the age of the second rise, the greater the risk of future obesity. Remember also that while BMI has a high correlation with relative fatness or leanness it is actually assessing the weight-to-height relationship: **this may give misleading results in boys who are very stocky and muscular who might appear obese on the BMI alone.**

BOYS
BMI CHART
(BIRTH - 20 YEARS)
United Kingdom cross-sectional reference data : 1997/1

Name..

NHS No. ☐☐☐ ☐☐☐ ☐☐☐☐

How to calculate BMI

Divide weight (kg) by square of length/height (m^2)
e.g. when weight = 25kg and length/height = 1.2m (120cm),
BMI = $25 \div (1.2 \times 1.2) = 17.4$

Date		Age	Length/Height	Weight	BMI	Initials
:	:	:	:	:	:	
:	:	:	:	:	:	
:	:	:	:	:	:	
:	:	:	:	:	:	
:	:	:	:	:	:	
:	:	:	:	:	:	

Body Mass Index (kg/m^2)

years

99.6th
98th
91st
75th
50th
25th
9th
2nd
0.4th

EDD

Data: 1990

Reference

Body Mass Index reference curves for the UK, 1990 (TJ Cole, JV Freeman, MA Preece) *Arch Dis Child* 1995; **73**: 25-29
Sex differences in weight in infancy (MA Preece, JV Freeman, TJ Cole) *BMJ* 1996; **313**: 1486

Manufacture 4 Mar. 01

Designed and Published by
© CHILD GROWTH FOUNDATION 1997/1
(Charity Reg. No 274325)
2 Mayfield Avenue,
London W4 1PW

Printed and Supplied by
HARLOW PRINTING LIMITED
Maxwell Street ◊ South Shields
Tyne & Wear ◊ NE33 4PU

The Milan Declaration

A statement on behalf of the European Association for the Study of Obesity made at the 9th European Congress on Obesity, Milan, Italy. June 3–6, 1999.

In view of the urgent need for action to deal with the epidemic of obesity and weight-related health issues, we members of the European Association for the Study of Obesity, with the support of others, call on governments and health agencies in Europe to:

- Recognize that overweight and obesity are major causes of ill health which present a huge social and economic burden to communities within Europe.

- Immediately begin the process of developing comprehensive national and European strategies for action on obesity which take into account the needs of each country, build upon existing initiatives and are based on sound evidence of benefit.

- Support continued research and analysis of the problem of overweight and obesity that will inform the development of improved obesity prevention and management strategies.

We also resolve to:

- Provide leadership, support and guidance to governments and agencies towards the development of coherent national and Europe-wide strategies for the prevention and management of overweight and obesity.

Signed by the presidents of national associations in membership of the European Association for the Study of Obesity

Index